every man's battle guide

**Weapons for the War
Against Sexual Temptation**

every man's
battle guide

Stephen Arterburn
Fred Stoeker with Mike Yorkey

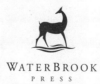

WATERBROOK
PRESS

EVERY MAN'S BATTLE GUIDE
PUBLISHED BY WATERBROOK PRESS
2375 Telstar Drive, Suite 160
Colorado Springs, Colorado 80920
A division of Random House, Inc.

ISBN 1-57856-736-X

Published in association with the literary agency of Alive Communications, Inc.,
7680 Goddard Street, Suite 200, Colorado Springs, CO 80920.

Printed in China
2003—First Edition

10 9 8 7 6 5 4 3 2 1

contents

introduction

The Word of God contains wonderful insight and apt reminders about God's standard regarding our sexual behavior and attitudes. Scripture offers a timeless source of encouragement that we can return to time and time again as we deal with issues of sexual integrity.

However, as we pointed out in our book *Every Man's Battle*, too many Christian men fail to crack open their Bibles on a regular basis, which means they are clueless when it comes to knowing God's standard for sexual purity. Others mix their own standards with God's Word with predictable results: messed-up lives, tons of heartache, and years of guilt that hangs around like a springtime cold.

Sexual integrity is an important topic in the Bible. Did you know we are commanded to avoid sexual impurity in *nearly every book* of the New Testament? The following fourteen New Testament scriptures, with references to sexual immorality highlighted in boldface type, demonstrate God's concern for our sexual purity:

> It is my judgment, therefore, that we should not make it difficult for the Gentiles who are turning to God. Instead we should write to them, telling them to abstain from food

polluted by idols, from **sexual immorality**, from the meat of strangled animals and from blood.

ACTS 15:19-20, NIV

So let us put aside the deeds of darkness and put on the armor of light. Let us behave decently, as in the daytime, not in orgies and drunkenness, not in **sexual immorality** and debauchery, not in dissension and jealousy.

ROMANS 13:12-13, NIV

But now I am writing you that you must not associate with anyone who calls himself a brother but is **sexually immoral** or greedy, an idolater or a slanderer, a drunkard or swindler. With such a man do not even eat.

1 CORINTHIANS 5:11, NIV

Flee from **sexual immorality**.

1 CORINTHIANS 6:18, NIV

I am afraid that when I come again my God will humble me before you, and I will be grieved over many who have sinned earlier and have not repented of the impurity, **sexual sin** and debauchery in which they have indulged.

2 CORINTHIANS 12:21, NIV

So I say, live by the Spirit, and you will not gratify the desires of the sinful nature.... The acts of the sinful

nature are obvious: **sexual immorality**, impurity and
debauchery…

GALATIANS 5:16,19, NIV

But among you there must not be even a hint of **sexual
immorality**, or of any kind of impurity, or of greed,
because these are improper for God's holy people. Nor
should there be obscenity, foolish talk or coarse joking,
which are out of place…

EPHESIANS 5:3-4, NIV

Put to death, therefore, whatever belongs to your earthly
nature: **sexual immorality**, impurity, lust, evil desires and
greed, which is idolatry. Because of these, the wrath of
God is coming.

COLOSSIANS 3:5-6, NIV

It is God's will that you should be sanctified: that you should
avoid **sexual immorality**; that each of you should learn to
control his own body in a way that is holy and honorable, not
in passionate lust like the heathen, who do not know God.

1 THESSALONIANS 4:3-5, NIV

See that no one is **sexually immoral**, or is godless like
Esau, who for a single meal sold his inheritance rights as
the oldest son.

HEBREWS 12:16, NIV

Marriage should be honored by all, and the marriage bed kept pure, for God will judge the adulterer and all the **sexually immoral**.

HEBREWS 13:4, NIV

Therefore, since Christ suffered in his body, arm your-selves.... For you have spent enough time in the past doing what pagans choose to do—living in debauchery, **lust**, drunkenness, orgies.

1 PETER 4:1,3, NIV

In a similar way, Sodom and Gomorrah and the surround-ing towns gave themselves up to **sexual immorality** and perversion. They serve as an example of those who suffer the punishment of eternal fire.

JUDE 7, NIV

Nevertheless, I [Jesus] have a few things against you: You have people there who hold to the teaching of Balaam, who taught Balak to entice the Israelites to sin by eating food sacrificed to idols and by committing **sexual immorality**.

REVELATION 2:14, NIV

Isn't that something? Fourteen of the twenty-seven books in the New Testament are represented here, which gives us an indication of how important God considers the topic of sexual integrity.

From the preceding set of scriptures, we can summarize His standard in the following words:

- It is holy and honorable to avoid sexual immorality because sexual immorality is an act of the sinful nature.
- We should not even eat or associate with another Christian who is sexually immoral.
- Even foolish talk and coarse joking are out of place for Christians.
- God says we have spent enough time living as the pagans do.
- Living in passionate lust is for those people who don't know God.
- Because of sexual immorality, the wrath of God is coming, along with punishment of eternal fire.
- Take this seriously! Flee sexual immorality!
- If you entice others into sexual immorality, Jesus Himself has something against you!

Clearly, God *does* expect us to live according to His standard. So the question becomes, How are you doing when your actions are measured against this standard? Or, asked another way, Do you have even a hint of sexual immorality in your life? If so, it's because some of these red flags are flapping in the breeze:

- Do you tell off-color jokes? Do you like to use double

entendres and make word plays with a double-sided sexual meaning?

- Do you channel-surf, hoping to catch a glimpse of something racy on television? Do you catch yourself watching voyeuristic shows?

- If a certain woman at your office calls in sick, do you feel a bit down in the dumps?

- Did your last hiring decision have more to do with a woman's body than with her résumé?

- Are you finding your wife to be less sexually satisfying than she once was?

- Do you have behaviors that you can't share with your wife?

- Do you have a secret compartment or private place you hide from your wife?

- Do you linger over lingerie ads and department store ad inserts in the newspaper on Sunday mornings?

- Do you watch women's figure skating or women's beach volleyball on television, although you have little sporting interest in the competition?

- Do you rent sexually explicit videos or go to movies where you can watch other people having sex?

- Do you turn on exercise shows just so you can enjoy those closeups of participants' breasts, rear ends, and inner thighs?

- Do you gaze at the glistening athletic bodies of joggers wearing tight nylon shorts?

- Do you admire the cute girl passing by, whistling to yourself and saying, "Nice rack"?
- Do you flirt—and know you're doing it?
- Do you communicate intimately with a person of the opposite sex in an Internet chat room?
- Do you fantasize about that woman from the chat room?
- When you are with your wife in bed, does another face flash across your mind?
- Do you daydream about other women?
- Do you dream hot scenes with other women at night?
- Do you think about old girlfriends when things aren't going well at home?
- When you are driving down the road with your wife, does your mind wander to that girl at work? Do you ever say things to yourself like, "I wonder if she ever thinks of me when she's not at work" or "I wonder what she is doing right now" or "I wonder if she is really happy with her husband"?
- Do you ever think, "God understands my sexuality. He knows how lonely I am. He knows I need this with her right now"? (A word to the wise: God doesn't think that way.)
- Did you chafe and get defensive or angry as you read through this list?

If any of these red flags are flying, then you have at least a hint of sexual immorality in your life, and we're encouraging you to do something about it.

Again, God *does* expect us to keep His standard, bearing in mind these three thoughts:

1. Yes, it's difficult.
2. No, it's not impossible.
3. And yes, you *can* do it.

You can do it because God has already given you the weapons you need. Those who have gone before you will tell you that soaking up God's Word on a regular basis is one of the best ways to prepare for battle. So consider this handy little volume your battle guide, a manual that details each of the defensive and offensive strategies God has laid out in His Word.

So what are you waiting for? Wouldn't today be a great day to begin? We welcome you to thumb through these exciting passages from Scripture and start building your arsenal in preparation for the inevitable attack. If you can commit some of these verses to memory, you'll be well on your way to winning Every Man's Battle.

you can depend on God

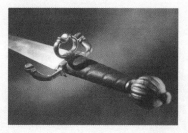

God's love for you is unconditional; it never changes. Before you were formed in the womb, He loved you. You're the apple of His eye. His love for you has no limits, and His love for you will never wane. When you couldn't put your porn magazines down, He still loved you. When you lay in the arms of another Saturday-night date, He still loved you. When you continued to ignore Him, He chased you desperately, aching to reach you before it was too late and your heart had hardened.

—adapted from *Every Young Man's Battle*

HIS WORDS ARE TRUE

Heaven and earth will pass away, but my words will never pass away.

MATTHEW 24:35, NIV

HIS LOVE IS TRUE

For God so loved the world, that he gave his only begotten Son, that whosoever believeth in him should not perish, but have everlasting life.

JOHN 3:16, KJV

God showed how much he loved us by sending his only Son into the world so that we might have eternal life through him. This is real love. It is not that we loved God, but that he loved us and sent his Son as a sacrifice to take away our sins.

1 JOHN 4:9-10, NLT

For I am persuaded, that neither death, nor life, nor angels, nor principalities, nor powers, nor things present, nor things to come, nor height, nor depth, nor any other creature, shall be able to separate us from the love of God, which is in Christ Jesus our Lord.

ROMANS 8:38-39, KJV

HIS COMMANDMENTS ARE BASED IN LOVE

For all God's words are right, and everything he does is worthy of our trust. He loves whatever is just and good; the earth is filled with his tender love.

PSALM 33:4-5, TLB

The words and promises of the Lord are pure words, like silver refined in an earthen furnace, purified seven times over.

PSALM 12:6, AMP

The LORD looks down from heaven
    and sees the whole human race.
From his throne he observes

all who live on the earth.
He made their hearts,
    so he understands everything they do.

PSALM 33:13-15, NLT

The statutes of the LORD are right, rejoicing the heart: the commandment of the LORD is pure, enlightening the eyes.

PSALM 19:8, KJV

God's work and commitment
on your behalf

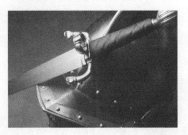

At Calvary, He purchased for you the freedom and authority to live in purity. That freedom and that authority are His gift to you through the presence of His Spirit, who took up residence within you when you gave your life to Christ. The freedom and authority are wrapped up in our new inner connection to His divine nature, which is the link that gives us His power and the fulfillment of His promises:

"His divine power has given us everything we need for life and godliness through our knowledge of him who called us by his own glory and goodness. Through these he has given us his very great and precious promises, so that through them you may participate in the divine nature and escape the corruption in the world caused by evil desires" (2 Peter 1:3-4, NIV).

—Every Man's Battle

CHRIST DIED FOR OUR SINS—AND WE STAND FORGIVEN

> He himself bore our sins in his body on the tree, so that we might die to sins and live for righteousness; by his wounds, you have been healed.
>
> 1 PETER 2:24, NIV

This includes you who were once so far away from God. You were his enemies, separated from him by your evil thoughts and actions, yet now he has brought you back as his friends. He has done this through his death on the cross in his own human body. As a result, he has brought you into the very presence of God, and you are holy and blameless as you stand before him without a single fault.

COLOSSIANS 1:21-22, NLT

And now you are free from your old master, sin; and you have become slaves to your new master, righteousness.

ROMANS 6:18, TLB

Remember that you were at that time separate from Christ, excluded from the commonwealth of Israel, and strangers to the covenants of promise, having no hope and without God in the world. But now in Christ Jesus you who formerly were far off have been brought near by the blood of Christ.

EPHESIANS 2:12-13, NASB

Always thanking the Father, who has enabled you to share the inheritance that belongs to God's holy people, who live in the light. For he has rescued us from the one who rules in the kingdom of darkness, and he has brought us into the Kingdom of his dear Son.

COLOSSIANS 1:12-13, NLT

For Christ is the end of the law, that every one who has faith may be justified.

ROMANS 10:4, RSV

GOD DESIGNED YOU FOR VICTORY

To God's elect…who have been chosen according to the foreknowledge of God the Father, through the sanctifying work of the Spirit, for obedience to Jesus Christ.

1 PETER 1:1-2, NIV

Long ago, even before he made the world, God loved us and chose us in Christ to be holy and without fault in his eyes.

EPHESIANS 1:4, NLT

In him, according to the purpose of him who accomplishes all things according to the counsel of his will, we who first hoped in Christ have been destined and appointed to live for the praise of his glory.

EPHESIANS 1:11-12, RSV

For we are his workmanship, created in Christ Jesus for good works, which God prepared beforehand, that we should walk in them.

EPHESIANS 2:10, RSV

GOD CLEARLY EXPRESSES HIS WILL FOR YOU

Each one of us has been manipulated by our sexual culture; each of us has made choices to sin. To varying degrees, each of us became ensnared by these choices, but we can overcome this affliction. Far too often, however, we ignore our own responsibility in this. We complain, "Well, *of course* I want to be free from impurity! I've been to the altar 433 times about it, haven't I? It just doesn't seem to be God's will to free me."

Not God's will? That's an offense to the character of God. Don't blame God.

God's will is for you to have sexual purity, though you may not think so since this hasn't been your constant experience. But He *has* made a provision for that purity.

—Every Man's Battle

It is God's will that you should be sanctified: that you should avoid sexual immorality; that each of you should learn to control his own body in a way that is holy and honorable.

1 THESSALONIANS 4:3-4, NIV

But be holy now in everything you do, just as the Lord is holy, who invited you to be his child. He himself has said, "You must be holy, for I am holy."

1 PETER 1:15-16, TLB

GOD IS WORKING TO TEACH YOU

For the grace of God that brings salvation has appeared to all men. It teaches us to say "No" to ungodliness and

worldly passions, and to live self-controlled, upright and
godly lives in this present age, while we wait for the blessed
hope…our great God and Savior, Jesus Christ.

TITUS 2:11-13, NIV

I will praise the LORD, who counsels me;
    even at night my heart instructs me.

PSALM 16:7, NIV

Good and upright is the LORD;
Therefore He instructs sinners in the way.
He leads the humble in justice,
And He teaches the humble His way.

PSALM 25:8-9, NASB

But when the Father sends the Counselor as my represen-
tative—and by the Counselor I mean the Holy Spirit—he
will teach you everything and will remind you of everything I myself have told you.

JOHN 14:26, NLT

GOD WANTS TO ENCOURAGE YOU

Surely he will never be shaken;
    a righteous man will be remembered forever.
He will have no fear of bad news;
    his heart is steadfast, trusting in the LORD.

His heart is secure, he will have no fear;
>   in the end he will look in triumph on his foes.

PSALM 112:6-8, NIV

You have made known to me the path of life;
>   you will fill me with joy in your presence,
>   with eternal pleasures at your right hand.

PSALM 16:11, NIV

Give your burdens to the LORD,
>   and he will take care of you.
>   He will not permit the godly to slip and fall.

PSALM 55:22, NLT

For I the LORD thy God will hold thy right hand, saying
unto thee, Fear not; I will help thee.

ISAIAH 41:13, KJV

GOD HAS PROMISED TO WALK WITH YOU

God is waiting for you. But He is not waiting by the altar, hoping you'll drop by and talk for a while. He is waiting for you to rise up and engage in the battle.

—*Every Man's Battle*

And surely I am with you always, to the very end of the age.

MATTHEW 28:20, NIV

When you pass through the waters, I will be with you;
And through the rivers, they will not overflow you.
When you walk through the fire, you will not be scorched,
Nor will the flame burn you.

Isaiah 43:2, nasb

Don't be afraid, for the Lord will go before you and will be
with you; he will not fail nor forsake you.

Deuteronomy 31:8, tlb

GOD IS WORKING TO SANCTIFY YOU

May the God of peace himself make you entirely pure and
devoted to God; and may your spirit and soul and body be
kept strong and blameless until that day when our Lord
Jesus Christ comes back again. God, who called you to
become his child, will do all this for you, just as he
promised.

1 Thessalonians 5:23-24, tlb

"Come now, let us argue this out," says the LORD. "No
matter how deep the stain of your sins, I can remove it. I
can make you as clean as freshly fallen snow. Even if you
are stained as red as crimson, I can make you as white
as wool."

Isaiah 1:18, nlt

Husbands, love your wives, just as Christ loved the church
and gave himself up for her to make her holy, cleansing her
by the washing with water through the word.

EPHESIANS 5:25-26, NIV

But if we walk in the light as He is in the light, we have
fellowship with one another, and the blood of Jesus Christ
His Son cleanses us from all sin.

1 JOHN 1:7, NKJV

And so we keep on praying for you, that our God will
make you the kind of children he wants to have—will
make you as good as you wish you could be!—rewarding
your faith with his power.

2 THESSALONIANS 1:11, TLB

And I am sure that God who began the good work within
you will keep right on helping you grow in his grace until
his task within you is finally finished on that day when
Jesus Christ returns.

PHILIPPIANS 1:6, TLB

GOD HAS PROMISED TO STRENGTHEN YOU

So do not fear, for I am with you;
    do not be dismayed, for I am your God.

I will strengthen you and help you;
> I will uphold you with my righteous right hand.

ISAIAH 41:10, NIV

Revive us, and we will call upon Your name.

PSALM 80:18, NASB

As a result, Christ will make your hearts strong, blameless, and holy when you stand before God our Father on that day when our Lord Jesus comes with all those who belong to him.

1 THESSALONIANS 3:13, NLT

Each time he said, "My gracious favor is all you need. My power works best in your weakness." So now I am glad to boast about my weaknesses, so that the power of Christ may work through me.

2 CORINTHIANS 12:9, NLT

GOD'S WORD IS AVAILABLE TO WORK IN YOU

And we will never stop thanking God for this: that when we preached to you, you didn't think of the words we spoke as being just our own, but you accepted what we said as the very Word of God—which, of course, it was—and it changed your lives when you believed it.

1 THESSALONIANS 2:13, TLB

For the word of God is living and active. Sharper than any double-edged sword, it penetrates even to dividing soul and spirit, joints and marrow; it judges the thoughts and attitudes of the heart.

HEBREWS 4:12, NIV

How can a young man cleanse his way?
By taking heed according to Your word.

PSALM 119:9, NKJV

The whole Bible was given to us by inspiration from God and is useful to teach us what is true and to make us realize what is wrong in our lives; it straightens us out and helps us do what is right. It is God's way of making us well prepared at every point, fully equipped to good to everyone.

2 TIMOTHY 3:16-17, TLB

GOD IS COMMITTED TO MAKING YOU HOLY

Our fathers disciplined us for a little while as they thought best; but God disciplines us for our good, that we may share in his holiness. No discipline seems pleasant at the time, but painful. Later on, however, it produces a harvest of righteousness and peace for those who have been trained by it.

HEBREWS 12:10-11, NIV

I continually discipline and punish everyone I love; so I
must punish you unless you turn from your indifference
and become enthusiastic about the things of God.

REVELATION 3:19, TLB

And have you quite forgotten the encouraging words God
spoke to you, his child? He said, "My son, don't be angry
when the Lord punishes you. Don't be discouraged when
he has to show you where you are wrong. For when he
punishes you, it proves that he loves you. When he whips
you, it proves you are really his child."

HEBREWS 12:5-6, TLB

GOD IS LISTENING TO JESUS, OUR ADVOCATE

Who shall bring a charge against God's elect? It is God
who justifies. Who is he who condemns? It is Christ who
died, and furthermore is also risen, who is even at the right
hand of God, who also makes intercession for us.

ROMANS 8:33-34, NKJV

Jesus lives forever.... Therefore he is able to save completely
those who come to God through him, because he always
lives to intercede for them.

HEBREWS 7:24,25, NIV

My little children, I am writing these things to you that you may not sin. And if anyone sins, we have an Advocate with the Father, Jesus Christ the righteous.

1 JOHN 2:1, NASB

victory can be yours

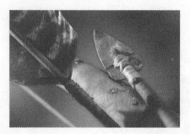

JESUS SHOWS THAT VICTORY IS POSSIBLE

Jesus' hands never touched a woman with dishonor, but Jesus said that lusting with the eyes is the same as touching. Given that Jesus is sinless, then it is true that Jesus not only never touched a woman with dishonor, He never even *looked* at a woman in dishonor. In this arena, Jesus is clearly our role model.

—adapted from *Every Man's Battle*

Christ, who suffered for you, is your example. Follow in his steps: He never sinned, never told a lie, never answered back when insulted… He personally carried the load of our sins in his own body when he died on the cross so that we can be finished with sin and live a good life from now on. For his wounds have healed ours!

1 PETER 2:21-24, TLB

Follow God's example in everything you do, because you are his dear children. Live a life filled with love for others, following the example of Christ, who loved you and gave himself as a sacrifice to take away your sins.

EPHESIANS 5:1-2, NLT

Therefore, when Christ came into the world, he said…
"Here I am—it is written about me in the scroll—

I have come to do your will, O God."

HEBREWS 10:5,7, NIV

But thanks be to God, which giveth us the victory through our Lord Jesus Christ.

1 CORINTHIANS 15:57, KJV

JOB SUCCEEDED IN THE BATTLE

His name was Job, a man who exemplifies the essential role model of sexual purity in Scripture. In the book of the Bible that tells his story, we see God bragging about Job to Satan: "Have you considered my servant Job? There is no one on earth like him; he is blameless and upright, a man who fears God and shuns evil" (Job 1:8, NIV).

Was God proud of Job? You bet! He applauded His servant's faithfulness in words of highest praise, and we should seek that same praise as well.

—adapted from *Every Man's Battle*

There lived in the land of Uz a man named Job—a good man who feared God and stayed away from evil.

JOB 1:1, TLB

If my heart has been enticed by a woman,
Or if I have lurked at my neighbor's door,

Then let my wife grind for another,
And let others bow down over her.
For that would be wickedness;
Yes, it would be iniquity deserving of
        judgment.

JOB 31:9-11, NKJV

YOU ARE NOT FIGHTING ALONE

We've known those who have failed in their battle for sexual purity, and we know some who have won. The difference? Those who won hated their impurity. They were going to war and were going to win—or die trying. Every resource was leveled upon the foe.

—Every Man's Battle

Therefore, since we are surrounded by such a great cloud
of witnesses, let us throw off everything that hinders and
the sin that so easily entangles, and let us run with perse-
verance the race marked out for us. Let us fix our eyes on
Jesus, the author and perfecter of our faith, who for the joy
set before him endured the cross, scorning its shame, and
sat down at the right hand of the throne of God. Consider
him who endured such opposition from sinful men, so
that you will not grow weary and lose heart.

HEBREWS 12:1-3, NIV

But I say, walk and live [habitually] in the [Holy] Spirit [responsive to and controlled and guided by the Spirit]; then you will certainly not gratify the cravings and desires of the flesh (of human nature without God).

GALATIANS 5:16, AMP

I pray that your hearts will be flooded with light so that you can understand the wonderful future he has promised to those he called. I want you to realize what a rich and glorious inheritance he has given to his people. I pray that you will begin to understand the incredible greatness of his power for us who believe him. This is the same mighty power that raised Christ from the dead and seated him in the place of honor at God's right hand in the heavenly realms.

EPHESIANS 1:18-20, NLT

I pray that from his glorious, unlimited resources he will give you mighty inner strength through his Holy Spirit.

EPHESIANS 3:16, NLT

you have weapons at your disposal

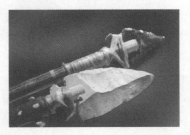

It's difficult to be victorious. We tell ourselves repeatedly that we want out, but our words are mere dandelion puffs, blowing about in the weakest breeze. Without resolute manhood girding our words, nothing happens. Here are some action items to help you decisively choose victory in the arena of sexual purity.

—adapted from *Every Man's Battle*

FASTING

In the spiritual realm, fasting breaks down every wall. In the physical realm, it strengthens our resolve. "I've suffered in my body through fasting in this battle—I won't lightly head off to that computer site again."

To succeed in your fasting, you are forced to answer the question, "Do I really want sexual freedom? Is sexual freedom more important than this next meal?" You'll be surprised how tough this question is to answer at the end of a day of fasting. Not eating will humble you, but this is good because fasting prioritizes your heart's passions. Suffering through fasting is transforming.

Since Christ suffered and underwent pain, you must have
the same attitude he did; you must be ready to suffer, too.
For remember, when your body suffers, sin loses its power,
and you won't be spending the rest of your life chasing
after evil desires but will be anxious to do the will of God.

1 PETER 4:1-2, TLB

> But as for me…I humbled my soul with fasting; and my
> prayer returned into mine own bosom.
>
> **PSALM 35:13**, KJV

PRAYER

When we pray, we aren't praying that He will decide to help us. He has already decided to help us. We are praying so that our hearts will change.

> For what great nation is there who has a god so near to
> them as the Lord our God is to us in all things for which
> we call upon Him?
>
> **DEUTERONOMY 4:7**, AMP

> Pray all the time. Ask God for anything in line with the
> Holy Spirit's wishes. Plead with him, reminding him of
> your needs, and keep praying earnestly for all Christians
> everywhere.
>
> **EPHESIANS 6:18**, TLB

> Be joyful in hope, patient in affliction, faithful in prayer.
>
> **ROMANS 12:12**, NIV

> Don't be weary in prayer; keep at it; watch for God's
> answers, and remember to be thankful when they come.
>
> **COLOSSIANS 4:2**, TLB

Be unceasing in prayer.

1 THESSALONIANS 5:17, AMP

But you, dear friends, build yourselves up in your most
holy faith and pray in the Holy Spirit.

JUDE 20, NIV

WORSHIP

What helps bring true intimacy with God quickly? Worship. We
were created to worship. Worship and praise bring intimacy with
the Lord and usher us quickly into His presence.

Chuck Swindoll once mentioned on his *Insight for Living* radio
broadcast that he never enters prayer without first entering worship.
That's a good place to start. You can memorize a few choruses and
hymns and sing them softly to the Lord before beginning prayer.

—adapted from *Every Young Man's Battle*

Yes, ascribe to the Lord
The glory due his name!
Bring an offering and come before him;
Worship the Lord when clothed with holiness!

1 CHRONICLES 16:29, TLB

Even if you suffer for doing what is right, God will reward
you for it. So don't be afraid and don't worry. Instead, you

must worship Christ as Lord of your life. And if you are asked about your Christian hope, always be ready to explain it. But you must do this in a gentle and respectful way. Keep your conscience clear. Then if people speak evil against you, they will be ashamed when they see what a good life you live because you belong to Christ. Remember, it is better to suffer for doing good, if that is what God wants, than to suffer for doing wrong!

1 PETER 3:14-17, NLT

Come, let us bow down in worship,
　　let us kneel before the LORD our Maker.

PSALM 95:6, NIV

You are worthy, O Lord our God,
　　to receive glory and honor and power.
For you created everything,
　　and it is for your pleasure that they exist and were
　　　　created.

REVELATION 4:11, NLT

MEDITATION

His heart of passion longs for you. Worship Him. He's the Creator of the universe, and He's *for* you.

—*Every Young Man's Battle*

But they delight in doing everything God wants them to
do, and day and night are always meditating on his laws
and thinking about ways to follow him more closely.

PSALM 1:2, TLB

This book of the law shall not depart from your mouth,
but you shall meditate on it day and night, so that you
may be careful to do according to all that is written in it;
for then you will make your way prosperous, and then you
will have success.

JOSHUA 1:8, NASB

On my bed I remember you;
    I think of you through the watches of the night.
Because you are my help,
    I sing in the shadow of your wings.

PSALM 63:6-7, NIV

YOUR SWORD

You'll need a good Bible verse to use as a sword and rallying
point.

Just one? It may be useful to memorize several verses of
Scripture about purity, as they work to eventually transform and
wash the mind. But in the cold-turkey, day-to-day fight against
impurity, having several verses committed to memory might be as
difficult as strapping on a hundred-pound backpack to engage in

hand-to-hand combat. That's why we recommend a single "attack verse," and we suggest the opening line of Job 31: "I have made a covenant with my eyes" [NIV].

When you fail and look at a sexy jogger, sharply say, "No, I've made a covenant with my eyes. I can't do that!" When you look at a busty billboard, say, "No, I've made a covenant with my eyes. I can't do that!" This action will be a quick dagger to the heart of your enemy.

—*Every Man's Battle*

And you will need the helmet of salvation and the sword of the Spirit—which is the Word of God.

EPHESIANS 6:17, TLB

For whatever God says to us is full of living power: it is sharper than the sharpest dagger, cutting swift and deep into our innermost thoughts and desires with all their parts, exposing us for what we really are.

HEBREWS 4:12, TLB

Your word is a lamp to my feet
    and a light for my path.

PSALM 119:105, NIV

Great peace have those who love Your law,
And nothing causes them to stumble.

PSALM 119:165, NKJV

> Your words were found, and I ate them; and Your words
> were to me a joy and the rejoicing of my heart, for I am
> called by Your name, O Lord God of hosts.
>
> JEREMIAH 15:16, AMP

YOUR SHIELD

Your shield—a protective verse that you can reflect on and draw strength from even when you aren't in the direct heat of battle—may be even more important than your sword, because it places temptation out of earshot.

We suggest this Scripture as your shield: "Flee from sexual immorality.... You are not your own; you were bought at a price. Therefore honor God with your body" (1 Corinthians 6:18-20, NIV).

It also helps to repeat this when facing sensual images or thoughts: "You have no right to look at that or think about it. You haven't the authority."

—adapted from *Every Man's Battle*

> In addition to all this, take up the shield of faith, with
> which you can extinguish all the flaming arrows of the evil
> one.
>
> EPHESIANS 6:16, NIV

you have to be accountable

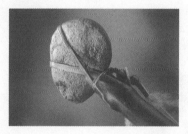

For many men fighting for sexual purity, an important step is finding accountability support in a men's Bible study group, from one or two other men serving as accountability partners, or by going into counseling.

For an accountability partner, you can enlist a male friend, perhaps someone older and well respected in the church, to encourage you in the heat of battle. The men's ministry at your church can also help you find someone who can pray for you and ask you the tough questions.

—adapted from _Every Man's Battle_

WE ARE ACCOUNTABLE TO GOD

What then shall I do when God rises up?
When he makes inquiry, what shall I answer
      him?

JOB 31:14, RSV

Arise, O LORD; O God, lift up Your hand.
Do not forget the afflicted.
Why has the wicked spurned God?
He has said to himself, "You will not require it."
You have seen it, for You have beheld mischief and
      vexation to take it into Your hand.
The unfortunate commits himself to You;
You have been the helper of the orphan.

Break the arm of the wicked and the evildoer,
Seek out his wickedness until You find none.

PSALM 10:12-15, NASB

He who deals wisely and heeds [God's] word and counsel
shall find good, and whoever leans on, trusts in, and
is confident in the Lord—happy, blessed, and fortunate
is he.

PROVERBS 16:20, AMP

If you sin without knowing what you're doing, God takes
that into account. But if you sin knowing full well what
you're doing, that's a different story entirely. Merely hearing God's law is a waste of time if you don't do what he
commands. Doing, not hearing, is what makes the difference with God.

ROMANS 2:12-13, MSG

But I say unto you, That every idle word that men shall
speak, they shall give account thereof in the day of
judgment.

MATTHEW 12:36, KJV

For this very reason, Christ died and returned to life so
that he might be the Lord of both the dead and the living.
You, then, why do you judge your brother? Or why do

you look down on your brother? For we will all stand
before God's judgment seat. It is written:

"'As surely as I live,' says the Lord,
'every knee will bow before me;
every tongue will confess to God.'"

So then, each of us will give an account of himself
to God.

ROMANS 14:9-12, NIV

The reverent and worshipful fear of the Lord prolongs
one's days, but the years of the wicked shall be made short.

PROVERBS 10:27, AMP

For God did not call us to be impure, but to live a holy
life. Therefore, he who rejects this instruction does not
reject man but God, who gives you his Holy Spirit.

1 THESSALONIANS 4:7-8, NIV

Nothing in all creation can hide from him. Everything is
naked and exposed before his eyes. This is the God to
whom we must explain all that we have done.

HEBREWS 4:13, NLT

You have had enough in the past of the evil things that
godless people enjoy—their immorality and lust, their
feasting and drunkenness and wild parties, and their
terrible worship of idols.

Of course, your former friends are very surprised when you no longer join them in the wicked things they do, and they say evil things about you. But just remember that they will have to face God, who will judge everyone, both the living and the dead.

1 PETER 4:3-5, NLT

And he called him, and said unto him, How is it that I hear this of thee? give an account of thy stewardship; for thou mayest be no longer steward.

LUKE 16:2, KJV

WHEN THE LORD DISCIPLINES YOU

My child, don't ignore it when the LORD disciplines you, and don't be discouraged when he corrects you. For the LORD corrects those he loves, just as a father corrects a child in whom he delights.

PROVERBS 3:11-12, NLT

Behold, happy is the man whom God corrects;
Therefore do not despise the chastening of the Almighty.

JOB 5:17, NKJV

The fear of the LORD is the beginning of knowledge;
Fools despise wisdom and instruction.

PROVERBS 1:7, NASB

Cease listening, my son, to discipline,
And you will stray from the words of knowledge.

PROVERBS 19:27, NASB

He who keeps instruction is in the way of life,
But he who refuses correction goes astray.

PROVERBS 10:17, NKJV

WE ARE ACCOUNTABLE TO ONE ANOTHER

My eyes will be on the faithful in the land,
    that they may dwell with me;
he whose walk is blameless
    will minister to me.

PSALM 101:6, NIV

It isn't our job to judge outsiders. But it certainly is our
job to judge and deal strongly with those who are members
of the church, and who are sinning in these ways. God alone
is the Judge of those on the outside. But you yourselves
must deal with this man and put him out of your church.

1 CORINTHIANS 5:12-13, TLB

Instruct a wise man and he will be wiser still;
    teach a righteous man and he will add to his learning.

PROVERBS 9:9, NIV

A rebuke goes deeper into a man of understanding
than a hundred blows into a fool.

PROVERBS 17:10, RSV

There are "friends" who destroy each other, but a real
friend sticks closer than a brother.

PROVERBS 18:24, NLT

Get all the advice and instruction you can, and be wise the
rest of your life.

PROVERBS 19:20, NLT

Open rebuke is better than hidden love!
Wounds from a friend are better than kisses from an
enemy!

PROVERBS 27:5-6, TLB

Then let us no more criticize and blame and pass judgment on one another, but rather decide and endeavor
never to put a stumbling block or an obstacle or a hin-
drance in the way of a brother.

ROMANS 14:13, AMP

Anyone who loves other Christians is living in the light
and does not cause anyone to stumble.

1 JOHN 2:10, NLT

LISTEN TO THOSE WHO HAVE GONE BEFORE YOU

Where there is no guidance the people fall,
But in abundance of counselors there is victory.

PROVERBS 11:14, NASB

Your testimonies also are my delight;
They are my counselors.

PSALM 119:24, NASB

Valid criticism is as treasured by the one who heeds it as
jewelry made from finest gold.

PROVERBS 25:12, NLT

Oil and perfume make the heart glad,
So a man's counsel is sweet to his friend.

PROVERBS 27:9, NASB

ACCOUNTABILITY IS VITAL TO YOUR SUCCESS

Without counsel purposes are disappointed; but in the
multitude of counsellors they are established.

PROVERBS 15:22, DARBY

The ear that hears the rebukes of life
Will abide among the wise.

PROVERBS 15:31, NKJV

From my experience, I know that fools who turn from
God may be successful for the moment, but then comes
sudden disaster.

JOB 5:3, NLT

But how quickly they [those who sin against God] dis-
appear from the face of the earth. Everything they own is
cursed. They leave no property for their children.

JOB 24:18, TLB

watch who you hang out with

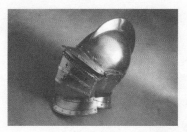

BEWARE OF THE TREACHERY OF OTHERS

For certain persons have crept in unnoticed, those who
were long beforehand marked out for this condemnation,
ungodly persons who turn the grace of our God into licen-
tiousness and deny our only Master and Lord, Jesus
Christ.

JUDE 4, NASB

Stay away from fools, for you won't find knowledge there.
The wise look ahead to see what is coming, but fools
deceive themselves.

PROVERBS 14:7-8, NLT

The wise man is glad to be instructed, but a self-sufficient
fool falls flat on his face.

PROVERBS 10:8, TLB

Men of perverse heart shall be far from me;
I will have nothing to do with evil.

PSALM 101:4, NIV

Fools think they need no advice, but the wise listen to others.

PROVERBS 12:15, NLT

But there were also false prophets in Israel, just as there
will be false teachers among you. They will cleverly teach

their destructive heresies about God and even turn against
their Master who bought them. Theirs will be a swift and
terrible end.

2 PETER 2:1, NLT

The crown of the wise is their riches,
But the folly of fools is foolishness.

PROVERBS 14:24, NASB

Good people are guided by their honesty; treacherous
people are destroyed by their dishonesty.

PROVERBS 11:3, NLT

The heart of the wise inclines to the right,
  but the heart of the fool to the left.

ECCLESIASTES 10:2, NIV

Their future is eternal destruction. Their god is their
appetite, they brag about shameful things, and all they
think about is this life here on earth.

PHILIPPIANS 3:19, NLT

INVEST YOUR TIME WITH MEN OF INTEGRITY

Follow the steps of good men instead, and stay on the
paths of the righteous. For only the upright will live in the
land, and those who have integrity will remain in it. But

the wicked will be removed from the land, and the treacherous will be destroyed.

PROVERBS 2:20-22, NLT

When I [Paul] wrote to you before, I told you not to associate with people who indulge in sexual sin.

1 CORINTHIANS 5:9, NLT

Although a wicked man commits a hundred crimes and
still lives a long time, I know that it will go better with
God-fearing men, who are reverent before God.

ECCLESIASTES 8:12, NIV

Blessed are the undefiled in the way,
Who walk in the law of the LORD!

PSALM 119:1, NKJV

For the wicked shall be cut off;
    but those who wait for the LORD shall possess the land.
The righteous shall possess the land,
    and dwell upon it for ever.

PSALM 37:9,29, RSV

LISTEN TO THE WISDOM OF YOUR COMMANDER

My son, do not forget my teaching,
But let your heart keep my commandments;

For length of days and years of life
And peace they will add to you.
Do not let kindness and truth leave you;
Bind them around your neck,
Write them on the tablet of your heart.
So you will find favor and good repute
In the sight of God and man.

PROVERBS 3:1-4, NASB

Sensible people keep their eyes glued on wisdom, but a
fool's eyes wander to the ends of the earth.

PROVERBS 17:24, NLT

The wise man's eyes are in his head, but the fool walks in
darkness.

ECCLESIASTES 2:14, NASB

For I command you today to love the LORD your God,
to walk in his ways, and to keep his commands, decrees
and laws; then you will live and increase, and the LORD
your God will bless you in the land you are entering to
possess.

DEUTERONOMY 30:16, NIV

With long life I will satisfy him,
And show him My salvation.

PSALM 91:16, NKJV

Hear, my son, and receive my sayings,
And the years of your life will be many.

PROVERBS 4:10, NKJV

The words of the wise heard in quiet are better than the
shouting of a ruler among fools.

ECCLESIASTES 9:17, RSV

how can something so wrong seem so right?

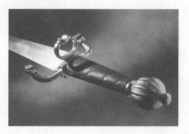

DON'T EMBRACE THE WISDOM OF THE WORLD

Claiming themselves to be wise without God, they became utter fools instead. And then, instead of worshiping the glorious, ever-living God, they took wood and stone and made idols for themselves, carving them to look like mere birds and animals and snakes and puny men.

ROMANS 1:22-23, TLB

Do not deceive yourselves. If any of you thinks he is wise by the standards of this age, he should become a "fool" so that he may become wise. For the wisdom of this world is foolishness in God's sight.

1 CORINTHIANS 3:18-19, NIV

WORLDLY DESIRES LEAD US AWAY FROM GOD

Whereas the object and purpose of our instruction and charge is love, which springs from a pure heart and a good (clear) conscience and sincere (unfeigned) faith.

But certain individuals have missed the mark on this very matter [and] have wandered away into vain arguments and discussions and purposeless talk.

1 TIMOTHY 1:5-6, AMP

But avoid worldly and empty chatter, for it will lead to further ungodliness, and their talk will spread like gangrene.

2 TIMOTHY 2:16-17, NASB

But when you follow your own wrong inclinations, your lives will produce these evil results: impure thoughts, eagerness for lustful pleasure,…envy, murder, drunkenness, wild parties, and all that sort of thing. Let me tell you again, as I have before, that anyone living that sort of life will not inherit the Kingdom of God.

GALATIANS 5:19,21, TLB

So the LORD replies to his people, "You love to wander far from me and do not follow in my paths. Now I will no longer accept you as my people. I will remember all your wickedness and will punish you for your sins."

JEREMIAH 14:10, NLT

So I tell you this, and insist on it in the Lord, that you must no longer live as the Gentiles do, in the futility of their thinking. They are darkened in their understanding and separated from the life of God because of the ignorance that is in them due to the hardening of their hearts. Having lost all sensitivity, they have given themselves over to sensuality so as to indulge in every kind of impurity, with a continual lust for more.

You, however, did not come to know Christ that way.…
You were taught, with regard to your former way of life, to
put off your old self, which is being corrupted by its deceitful
desires; to be made new in the attitude of your minds; and to
put on the new self, created to be like God in true righteousness and holiness.

EPHESIANS 4:17-24, NIV

WE HAVE FREEDOM TO LIVE MORALLY, NOT FREEDOM TO SIN

For, brethren, ye have been called unto liberty; only use
not liberty for an occasion to the flesh, but by love serve
one another.

GALATIANS 5:13, KJV

Act as free men, and do not use your freedom as a covering
for evil, but use it as bondslaves of God.

1 PETER 2:16, NASB

For they mouth empty, boastful words and, by appealing
to the lustful desires of sinful human nature, they entice
people who are just escaping from those who live in error.
They promise them freedom, while they themselves are
slaves of depravity—for a man is a slave to whatever has
mastered him.

2 PETER 2:18-19, NIV

EXAMINE YOURSELF TO SEE WHERE YOU ARE

If anyone thinks himself to be something, when he is
nothing, he deceives himself. But let each one examine his
own work, and then he will have rejoicing in himself
alone, and not in another.

GALATIANS 6:3-4, NKJV

Examine yourselves to see whether you are in the faith; test
yourselves. Do you not realize that Christ Jesus is in you—
unless, of course, you fail the test?

2 CORINTHIANS 13:5, NIV

Let us examine our ways and test them,
        and let us return to the LORD.

LAMENTATIONS 3:40, NIV

If you live according to the flesh you will die; but if by the
Spirit you put to death the deeds of the body, you will live.

ROMANS 8:13, NKJV

Beloved, if our heart does not condemn us, we have confidence before God; and whatever we ask we receive from
Him, because we keep His commandments and do the
things that are pleasing in His sight.

1 JOHN 3:21-22, NASB

TURN YOUR THOUGHTS AROUND

But take heed to yourselves, lest your hearts be weighed
down with carousing, drunkenness, and cares of this life,
and that Day come on you unexpectedly.

LUKE 21:34, NKJV

And now a personal but most urgent matter; I write in the
gentle but firm spirit of Christ. I hear that I'm being
painted as cringing and wishy-washy when I'm with you,
but harsh and demanding when at a safe distance writing
letters. Please don't force me to take a hard line when I'm
present with you. Don't think that I'll hesitate a single
minute to stand up to those who say I'm an unprincipled
opportunist. Then they'll have to eat their words.

The world is unprincipled. It's dog-eat-dog out there!
The world doesn't fight fair. But we don't live or fight our
battles that way—never have and never will. The tools of
our trade aren't for marketing or manipulation, but they
are for demolishing that entire massively corrupt culture.
We use our powerful God-tools for smashing warped
philosophies, tearing down barriers erected against the
truth of God, fitting every loose thought and emotion and
impulse into the structure of life shaped by Christ. Our
tools are ready at hand for clearing the ground of every
obstruction and building lives of obedience into maturity.

2 CORINTHIANS 10:1-6, MSG

Be anxious for nothing, but in everything by prayer and supplication, with thanksgiving, let your requests be made known to God; and the peace of God, which surpasses all understanding, will guard your hearts and minds through Christ Jesus.

PHILIPPIANS 4:6-8, NKJV

And so, dear brothers and sisters who belong to God and are bound for heaven, think about this Jesus whom we declare to be God's Messenger and High Priest.

HEBREWS 3:1, NLT

Keep your eyes on Jesus, our leader and instructor. He was willing to die a shameful death on the cross because of the joy he knew would be his afterwards; and now he sits in the place of honor by the throne of God. If you want to keep from becoming fainthearted and weary, think about his patience as sinful men did such terrible things to him.

HEBREWS 12:2-3, TLB

weighing the cost of
your choices

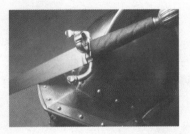

Mixture can destroy a people. When the Israelites left Egypt and were led to the Promised Land, God told them to cross the Jordan River and destroy every evil thing in their new homeland. That meant killing all the heathen people and crushing their gods to powder. God warned them that if they failed to do this, their culture would "mix" with the pagans and they would adopt their depraved practices.

But the Israelites were not careful to destroy everything. They found it easier and easier to stop short. In time, the things and people left undestroyed became a snare. The Israelites became adulterous in their relationship to God and repeatedly turned their backs on Him.

As promised, He removed them from their land. But just before the destruction of Jerusalem and the final deportation of her inhabitants, God prophesied this about His people in their coming captivity: "Then in the nations where they have been carried captive, those who escape will remember me—how I have been grieved by their adulterous hearts, which have turned away from me, and by their eyes, which have lusted after their idols. They will *loathe themselves* for the evil they have done" (Ezekiel 6:9, NIV).

When we entered the Promised Land of our salvation, we were told to eliminate every hint of sexual immorality in our lives. Since entering that land, have you failed to crush sexual sin? Every hint of it? If not, you need to heed God's warnings.

—adapted from *Every Man's Battle*

GOD WILL NOT IGNORE SIN

This also is God's will: that you never cheat in this matter by taking another man's wife, because the Lord will punish you terribly for this, as we have solemnly told you before.

1 THESSALONIANS 4:6, TLB

My son, be attentive to my wisdom,
    incline your ear to my understanding;
that you may keep discretion,
    and your lips may guard knowledge.
For the lips of a loose woman drip honey,
    and her speech is smoother than oil;
but in the end she is bitter as wormwood,
    sharp as a two-edged sword.

PROVERBS 5:1-4, RSV

I show this unfailing love to many thousands by forgiving every kind of sin and rebellion. Even so I do not leave sin unpunished, but I punish the children for the sins of their parents to the third and fourth generations.

EXODUS 34:7, NLT

The LORD is slow to anger and great in power,
And the LORD will by no means leave the guilty
    unpunished.

In whirlwind and storm is His way,
And clouds are the dust beneath His feet.

NAHUM 1:3, NASB

YOUR CHOICES WILL HAVE LASTING CONSEQUENCES

There is severe discipline for him who forsakes God's way;
and he who hates reproof will die [physically, morally, and
spiritually].

PROVERBS 15:10, AMP

The memory of the just is blessed: but the name of the
wicked shall rot.

PROVERBS 10:7, KJV

"You are proud because you live in those high, inaccessible
cliffs. 'Who can ever reach us way up here!' you boast.
Don't fool yourselves! Although you soar as high as eagles,
and build your nest among the stars, I will bring you
plummeting down," says the Lord.

OBADIAH 3-4, TLB

But the good man walks along in the ever-brightening
light of God's favor; the dawn gives way to morning splen-
dor, while the evil man gropes and stumbles in the dark.

Listen, son of mine, to what I say. Listen carefully.
Keep these thoughts ever in mind; let them penetrate deep

within your heart, for they will mean real life for you and
radiant health.

PROVERBS 4:18-22, TLB

Now your sins will be exposed for all to see; ashamed and
defenseless, you will be cut off forever.... Your acts will
boomerang upon your heads.

OBADIAH 10,15, TLB

Disaster will come upon you,
 and you will not know how to conjure it away.
A calamity will fall upon you
 that you cannot ward off with a ransom;
a catastrophe you cannot foresee
 will suddenly come upon you.

ISAIAH 47:11, NIV

[Folly] says, "Stolen water is refreshing; food eaten in secret
tastes the best!" But the men don't realize that her former
guests are now in the grave.

PROVERBS 9:17-18, NLT

LYING ONLY MAKES THINGS WORSE

A false witness [is one] who speaks lies,
And one who sows discord among brethren.

PROVERBS 6:19, NKJV

Right and just lips are the delight of a king, and he loves
him who speaks what is right.

PROVERBS 16:13, AMP

A false witness will not go unpunished,
And he who speaks lies will not escape.

PROVERBS 19:5, NKJV

I will not allow deceivers to serve me,
and liars will not be allowed to enter my presence.

PSALM 101:7, NLT

You shall not bear a false report; do not join your hand
with a wicked man to be a malicious witness.

EXODUS 23:1, NASB

A false witness shall be punished, and a liar shall be caught.

PROVERBS 19:9, TLB

With his mouth the godless destroys his neighbor,
but through knowledge the righteous escape.

PROVERBS 11:9, NIV

The desire of a man is his kindness: and a poor man is
better than a liar.

PROVERBS 19:22, KJV

WHEN YOU THINK GOD DOESN'T SEE YOUR SECRET SIN

The LORD is watching everywhere, keeping his eye on both the evil and the good.

PROVERBS 15:3, NLT

The depths of hell are open to God's knowledge. How much more the hearts of all mankind!

PROVERBS 15:11, TLB

For the eyes of the LORD move to and fro throughout the earth that He may strongly support those whose heart is completely His.

2 CHRONICLES 16:9, NASB

For My eyes are on all their ways; they are not hidden from My face, nor is their iniquity concealed from My eyes.

JEREMIAH 16:17, NASB

You have placed our iniquities before You,
Our secret sins in the light of Your presence.

PSALM 90:8, NASB

Do not keep talking so proudly
    or let your mouth speak such arrogance,

for the LORD is a God who knows,
and by him deeds are weighed.

1 SAMUEL 2:3, NIV

He reveals deep and secret things;
He knows what is in the darkness.

DANIEL 2:22, NKJV

WHAT DOES GOD THINK OF YOUR CHOICES?

The LORD detests the way of the wicked
but he loves those who pursue righteousness.

PROVERBS 15:9, NIV

The LORD preserves knowledge, but he ruins the plans of
the deceitful.

PROVERBS 22:12, NLT

The LORD is far from the wicked: but he heareth the
prayer of the righteous.

PROVERBS 15:29, KJV

Again and again I sent all my servants the prophets to you.
They said, "Each of you must turn from your wicked ways
and reform your actions; do not follow other gods to serve
them. Then you will live in the land I have given to you

and your fathers." But you have not paid attention or listened to me.

JEREMIAH 35:15, NIV

For you first, God raised up His Servant and sent Him to bless you by turning every one of you from your wicked ways.

ACTS 3:26, NASB

The tongues of those who are upright and in right standing with God are as choice silver; the minds of those who are wicked and out of harmony with God are of little value.

PROVERBS 10:20, AMP

Do you think, asks the Sovereign LORD, that I like to see wicked people die? Of course not! I only want them to turn from their wicked ways and live.

EZEKIEL 18:23, NLT

ANTICIPATE THE OUTCOME

Do not be envious of evil men,
Nor desire to be with them....
Do not fret because of evildoers
Or be envious of the wicked;

For there will be no future for the evil man;
The lamp of the wicked will be put out.

PROVERBS 24:1,19-20, NASB

For what profit is it to a man if he gains the whole world,
and is himself destroyed or lost?

LUKE 9:25, NKJV

The crooked heart will not prosper; the twisted tongue
tumbles into trouble.

PROVERBS 17:20, NLT

Thorns and snares are in the way of the obstinate and will-
ful; he who guards himself will be far from them.

PROVERBS 22:5, AMP

You're still teaching Sunday school, still singing in the choir, still
supporting your family. You've been faithful to your wife...well, at
least you haven't had an actual physical affair. You're getting
ahead in life, living in a nice home with nice cars and nice clothes
and a nice future. *People look to me as an example,* you reason.
I'm okay.

Yet privately, your conscience dims until you can't quite tell
what's right or wrong anymore. You're choking in the sexual prison
you've made, wondering where the promises of God have gone.
You spin in the same sinful cycles, year after year.

And nagging you is the worship. The prayer times. The distance, always the distance from God.

—*Every Man's Battle*

Then they will call upon me, but I will not answer;
    they will seek me diligently but will not find me.
Because they hated knowledge
    and did not choose the fear of the LORD,
would have none of my counsel,
    and despised all my reproof,
therefore they shall eat the fruit of their way
    and be sated with their own devices.

PROVERBS 1:28-31, RSV

If I have made gold my trust,
    or called fine gold my confidence;
if I have rejoiced because my wealth was great,
    or because my hand had gotten much;
if I have looked at the sun when it shone,
    or the moon moving in splendor,
and my heart has been secretly enticed,
    and my mouth has kissed my hand;
this also would be an iniquity to be punished
        by the judges,
    for I should have been false to God above.

JOB 31:24-28, RSV

For, behold, those who are far from You will perish;
You have destroyed all those who are unfaithful to You.

PSALM 73:27, NASB

And the heathen shall know that the house of Israel went
into captivity for their iniquity: because they trespassed
against me, therefore hid I my face from them, and gave
them into the hand of their enemies: so fell they all by
the sword.

EZEKIEL 39:23, KJV

I want you to be merciful; I don't want your sacrifices. I
want you to know God; that's more important than burnt
offerings.

But like Adam, you broke my covenant and rebelled
against me.

HOSEA 6:6-7, NLT

You adulterous people, don't you know that friendship with
the world is hatred toward God? Anyone who chooses to
be a friend of the world becomes an enemy of God.

JAMES 4:4, NIV

SIN WILL HARDEN YOUR HEART

He who hardens his heart will fall into calamity.

PROVERBS 28:14, NKJV

I don't understand myself at all, for I really want to do what is right, but I don't do it. Instead, I do the very thing I hate. I know perfectly well that what I am doing is wrong, and my bad conscience shows that I agree that the law is good. But I can't help myself, because it is sin inside me that makes me do these evil things.

ROMANS 7:15, NLT

God's owner's manual regarding sexual conduct

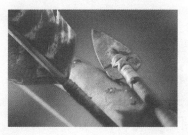

The world's sophisticates find God's standards ridiculous and con-fining. We live in a world awash with sensual images available twenty-four hours a day in a variety of mediums: print, television, videos, the Internet—even phones. But God offers us freedom from the slavery of sin through the cross of Christ, and He created our eyes and minds with an ability to be trained and controlled. We simply have to stand up and walk by His power in the right path, a path He has clearly marked out for us in His "owner's manual" for sexual conduct.

—adapted from *Every Man's Battle*

PURITY KEEPS LIFE RUNNING SMOOTHLY

He who loves purity of heart
And has grace on his lips,
The king will be his friend.

PROVERBS 22:11, NKJV

Who may ascend into the hill of the LORD?
Or who may stand in His holy place?
He who has clean hands and a pure heart,
Who has not lifted up his soul to an idol,
Nor sworn deceitfully.
He shall receive blessing from the LORD,
And righteousness from the God of his salvation.

PSALM 24:3-5, NKJV

But you are not in darkness, brethren, for that day to surprise you like a thief. For you are all sons of light and sons of the day; we are not of the night or of darkness. So then let us not sleep, as others do, but let us keep awake and be sober. For those who sleep sleep at night, and those who get drunk are drunk at night. But, since we belong to the day, let us be sober, and put on the breastplate of faith and love, and for a helmet the hope of salvation.

1 Thessalonians 5:4-8, rsv

WARNINGS AGAINST SEXUAL IMMORALITY

And He said, "What comes out of a man, that defiles a man. For from within, out of the heart of men, proceed evil thoughts, adulteries, fornications, [and] murders."

Mark 7:20-21, nkjv

Put to death therefore what is earthly in you: fornication, impurity, passion, evil desire, and covetousness, which is idolatry.

On account of these the wrath of God is coming.

Colossians 3:5-6, rsv

Treasures gained by wickedness do not profit,
    but righteousness delivers from death.

Proverbs 10:2, rsv

Do not be deceived; God is not mocked, for whatever a
man sows, that he will also reap.

GALATIANS 6:7, RSV

We are all infected and impure with sin. When we proudly
display our righteous deeds, we find they are but filthy
rags. Like autumn leaves, we wither and fall. And our sins,
like the wind, sweep us away.

ISAIAH 64:6, NLT

Wisdom is better than weapons of war, but one sinner
destroys much good.

ECCLESIASTES 9:18, RSV

Beloved, I implore you as aliens and strangers and exiles
[in this world] to abstain from the sensual urges (the evil
desires, the passions of the flesh, your lower nature) that
wage war against the soul.

1 PETER 2:11, AMP

MANUFACTURER'S WARNINGS REGARDING SEX

The LORD said to Moses, "Speak to the Israelites and say
to them: 'I am the LORD your God. You must not do as
they do in Egypt, where you used to live, and you must
not do as they do in the land of Canaan, where I am
bringing you. Do not follow their practices. You must

obey my laws and be careful to follow my decrees. I am the LORD your God. Keep my decrees and laws, for the man who obeys them will live by them. I am the LORD.

"'No one is to approach any close relative to have sexual relations. I am the LORD.

"'Do not dishonor your father by having sexual relations with your mother. She is your mother; do not have relations with her.

"'Do not have sexual relations with your father's wife; that would dishonor your father.

"'Do not have sexual relations with your sister, either your father's daughter or your mother's daughter, whether she was born in the same home or elsewhere.

"'Do not have sexual relations with your son's daughter or your daughter's daughter; that would dishonor you.

"'Do not have sexual relations with the daughter of your father's wife, born to your father; she is your sister.

"'Do not have sexual relations with your father's sister; she is your father's close relative.

"'Do not have sexual relations with your mother's sister, because she is your mother's close relative.

"'Do not dishonor your father's brother by approaching his wife to have sexual relations; she is your aunt.

"'Do not have sexual relations with your daughter-in-law. She is your son's wife; do not have relations with her.

"'Do not have sexual relations with your brother's wife; that would dishonor your brother.

"'Do not have sexual relations with both a woman and her daughter. Do not have sexual relations with either her son's daughter or her daughter's daughter; they are her close relatives. That is wickedness.

"'Do not take your wife's sister as a rival wife and have sexual relations with her while your wife is living.

"'Do not approach a woman to have sexual relations during the uncleanness of her monthly period.

"'Do not have sexual relations with your neighbor's wife and defile yourself with her.

"'Do not give any of your children to be sacrificed to Molech, for you must not profane the name of your God. I am the LORD.

"'Do not lie with a man as one lies with a woman; that is detestable.

"'Do not have sexual relations with an animal and defile yourself with it. A woman must not present herself to an animal to have sexual relations with it; that is a perversion.

"'Do not defile yourselves in any of these ways, because this is how the nations that I am going to drive out before you became defiled. Even the land was defiled; so I punished it for its sin, and the land vomited out its inhabitants. But you must keep my decrees and my laws. The native-born and the aliens living among you must not do any of these detestable things, for all these things were done by the people who lived in the land before you, and the land became defiled. And if you defile the land, it will vomit you out as it vomited out the nations that were before you.

"'Everyone who does any of these detestable things—such persons must be cut off from their people. Keep my requirements and do not follow any of the detestable customs that were practiced before you came and do not defile yourselves with them. I am the LORD your God.'"

LEVITICUS 18:1-29, NIV

DON'T ALLOW SEXUAL PLEASURE TO BECOME AN IDOL

You shall have no other gods before or besides Me.

EXODUS 20:3, AMP

You shall not follow other gods, any of the gods of the peoples who surround you.

DEUTERONOMY 6:14, NASB

Don't anger me by worshiping idols; but if you are true to me, then I'll not harm you.

JEREMIAH 25:6, TLB

It shall come about if you ever forget the LORD your God, and go after other gods and serve them and worship them, I testify against you today that you will surely perish.

DEUTERONOMY 8:19, NASB

your wife can be
your comrade in arms

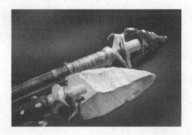

Your goal is sexual purity. Here's a good working definition of it—good because of its simplicity: *You are sexually pure when no sexual gratification comes from anyone or anything but your wife.* Purity means stopping sexual gratification that comes to us from outside our marriage.

—Every Man's Battle

YOUR WIFE IS A GIFT FROM GOD

Drink water from your own well—share your love only with your wife. Why spill the water of your springs in public, having sex with just anyone? You should reserve it for yourselves. Don't share it with strangers.

PROVERBS 5:15-17, NLT

How beautiful you are, my darling!
   Oh, how beautiful!
   Your eyes behind your veil are doves.
Your hair is like a flock of goats
   descending from Mount Gilead.
Your teeth are like a flock of sheep just shorn,
   coming up from the washing.
Each has its twin;
   not one of them is alone.
Your lips are like a scarlet ribbon;
   your mouth is lovely.
Your temples behind your veil

are like the halves of a pomegranate.
Your neck is like the tower of David,
    built with elegance;
on it hang a thousand shields,
    all of them shields of warriors.
Your two breasts are like two fawns,
    like twin fawns of a gazelle
    that browse among the lilies.

SONG OF SONGS 4:1-5, NIV

SEX IN A FAITHFUL MARRIAGE IS GOD'S PERFECT DESIGN

So God created people in his own image;
    God patterned them after himself;
    male and female he created them.
God blessed them and told them, "Multiply and fill
        the earth…"

GENESIS 1:27-28, NLT

The Lord God said, "It isn't good for man to be alone; I will
make a companion for him, a helper suited to his needs."

GENESIS 2:18, TLB

Therefore a man leaves his father and his mother and
cleaves to his wife, and they become one flesh. And the
man and his wife were both naked, and were not ashamed.

GENESIS 2:24-26, RSV

Adam slept with his wife, Eve, and she became pregnant. When the time came, she gave birth to Cain, and she said, "With the LORD's help, I have brought forth a man!"

GENESIS 4:1, NLT

And he answered and said unto them, Have ye not read, that he which made them at the beginning made them male and female, and said, For this cause shall a man leave father and mother, and shall cleave to his wife: and they twain shall be one flesh? Wherefore they are no more twain, but one flesh. What therefore God hath joined together, let not man put asunder.

MATTHEW 19:4-6, KJV

The husband should not deprive his wife of sexual intimacy, which is her right as a married woman, nor should the wife deprive her husband. The wife gives authority over her body to her husband, and the husband also gives authority over his body to his wife. So do not deprive each other of sexual relations. The only exception to this rule would be the agreement of both husband and wife to refrain from sexual intimacy for a limited time, so they can give themselves more completely to prayer. Afterward they should come together again so that Satan won't be able to tempt them because of their lack of self-control.

1 CORINTHIANS 7:3-5, NLT

YOU'RE IN THIS BATTLE TOGETHER

If anyone says, "I am living in the light," but hates a Christian brother or sister, that person is still living in darkness. Anyone who loves other Christians is living in the light and does not cause anyone to stumble. Anyone who hates a Christian brother or sister is living and walking in darkness. Such a person is lost, having been blinded by the darkness.

1 JOHN 2:9-11, NLT

Bear one another's burdens, and so fulfill the law of Christ.

GALATIANS 6:2, NKJV

Is there any encouragement from belonging to Christ? Any comfort from his love? Any fellowship together in the Spirit? Are your hearts tender and sympathetic? Then make me truly happy by agreeing wholeheartedly with each other, loving one another, and working together with one heart and purpose.

Don't be selfish; don't live to make a good impression on others. Be humble, thinking of others as better than yourself. Don't think only about your own affairs, but be interested in others, too, and what they are doing.

PHILIPPIANS 2:1-4, NLT

THE BENEFITS OF A GOOD WIFE

Whether your wife is wide or narrow or lumpy or smooth, when you focus your full attention on "your fountain," she'll become ever more beautiful to you. Her weak points will become sexy because they're yours and yours alone. They're all you have, and you can cherish them and let them fulfill you.

Maybe this shouldn't surprise us so much. After all, standards of beauty are not fixed. In centuries past, the great master painters depicted heavy, rounded women as the ultimate beauty. In the 1920s, thin, flat-chested women reigned. In the 1960s, the full-breasted, voluptuous girls were queen. In the 1980s and 1990s, muscled, glistening athletic women ignited us. Men adapt to each time period, their tastes formed by what they view, and the same will happen in this new millennium.

If you limit your eyes to your wife only, your own tastes will adapt to what you're viewing. Your wife's strengths *and* weaknesses will become your tastes. Eventually, she'll be beyond comparison in your eyes.

—*Every Man's Battle*

Let your wife be a fountain of blessing for you. Rejoice in the wife of your youth. She is a loving doe, a graceful deer. Let her breasts satisfy you always. May you always be captivated by her love.

PROVERBS 5:18-19, NLT

Enjoy life with the wife whom you love, all the days of
your vain life which he has given you under the sun,
because that is your portion in life and in your toil at
which you toil under the sun.

ECCLESIASTES 9:9, RSV

House and wealth are an inheritance from fathers,
But a prudent wife is from the LORD.

PROVERBS 19:14, NASB

He who finds a wife finds a good thing,
And obtains favor from the LORD.

PROVERBS 18:22, NKJV

My lover is to me a cluster of henna blossoms
    from the vineyards of En Gedi.
How beautiful you are, my darling!
    Oh, how beautiful!
    Your eyes are doves.

SONG OF SONGS 1:14-15, NIV

how to avoid being captured by the enemy

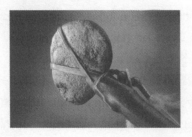

A search for mere excellence is an inadequate approach to God, leaving us vulnerable to snare after snare. Our only hope is obedience.

If we don't kill every hint of immorality, we'll be captured by our tendency as males to draw sexual gratification and chemical highs through our eyes.

—*Every Man's Battle*

LEARN FROM THE MISTAKES OF OTHERS

One day Dinah, Leah's daughter, went to visit some of the young women who lived in the area. But when the local prince, Shechem son of Hamor the Hivite, saw her, he took her and raped her.... Word soon reached Jacob that his daughter had been defiled, but his sons were out in the fields herding cattle so he did nothing until they returned. Meanwhile, Hamor, Shechem's father, came out to discuss the matter with Jacob. He arrived just as Jacob's sons were coming in from the fields. They were shocked and furious that their sister had been raped. Shechem had done a disgraceful thing against Jacob's family, a thing that should never have been done.

But three days later…two of Dinah's brothers, Simeon and Levi, took their swords, entered the town without opposition, and slaughtered every man there, including Hamor and Shechem. They rescued Dinah from Shechem's house and returned to their camp. Then all of Jacob's sons plundered the town because their sister had been defiled there. They seized all the flocks and herds and donkeys—everything they could lay their hands on, both inside the town and outside in the fields.

GENESIS 34:1-2,5-7,25-28, NLT

In a similar way, Sodom and Gomorrah and the surrounding towns gave themselves up to sexual immorality and perversion. They serve as an example of those who suffer the punishment of eternal fire.

JUDE 7, NIV

BE AWARE OF THE CONSEQUENCES OF SIN

So God let them go ahead and do whatever shameful things their hearts desired. As a result, they did vile and degrading things with each other's bodies....

And the men, instead of having normal sexual relationships with women, burned with lust for each other. Men did shameful things with other men and, as a result, suffered within themselves the penalty they so richly deserved.

ROMANS 1:24,27, NLT

Even a child is known by his deeds,
By whether what he does is pure and right.

PROVERBS 20:11, NKJV

I said to myself, "In due season God will judge everything man does, both good and bad."

ECCLESIASTES 3:17, TLB

Keep to a path far from her,
    do not go near the door of her house,
lest you give your best strength to others
    and your years to one who is cruel,
lest strangers feast on your wealth
    and your toil enrich another man's house.
At the end of your life you will groan,
    when your flesh and body are spent.
You will say, "How I hated discipline!
    How my heart spurned correction!
I would not obey my teachers
    or listen to my instructors.
I have come to the brink of utter ruin
    in the midst of the whole assembly."

PROVERBS 5:8-14, NIV

YOU CAN RESIST THE ENEMY

So put to death the sinful, earthly things lurking within you. Have nothing to do with sexual sin, impurity, lust, and shameful desires.

COLOSSIANS 3:5, NLT

Do you not know that your bodies are members of Christ?
Shall I therefore take the members of Christ and make
them members of a prostitute? Never! Do you not know
that he who joins himself to a prostitute becomes one
body with her? For, as it is written, "The two shall become
one flesh." But he who is united to the Lord becomes
one spirit with him. Shun immorality. Every other sin
which a man commits is outside the body; but the
immoral man sins against his own body. Do you not
know that your body is a temple of the Holy Spirit within
you, which you have from God? You are not your own;
you were bought with a price. So glorify God in your
body.

1 CORINTHIANS 6:15-20, RSV

Do not yield your members to sin as instruments of
wickedness, but yield yourselves to God as men who
have been brought from death to life, and your members
to God as instruments of righteousness.

ROMANS 6:13, RSV

Therefore, I urge you, brothers, in view of God's mercy, to
offer your bodies as living sacrifices, holy and pleasing to
God—this is your spiritual act of worship. Do not conform any longer to the pattern of this world, but be transformed by the renewing of your mind. Then you will be

able to test and approve what God's will is—his good,
pleasing and perfect will.

ROMANS 12:1-2, NIV

TURN TO YOUR SUPPORT TEAM

The human body has many parts, but the many parts
make up only one body. So it is with the body of Christ.
Some of us are Jews, some are Gentiles, some are slaves,
and some are free. But we have all been baptized into
Christ's body by one Spirit, and we have all received the
same Spirit.

Yes, the body has many different parts, not just one
part. If the foot says, "I am not a part of the body because
I am not a hand," that does not make it any less a part of
the body. And if the ear says, "I am not part of the body
because I am only an ear and not an eye," would that
make it any less a part of the body? Suppose the whole
body were an eye—then how would you hear? Or if your
whole body were just one big ear, how could you smell
anything?

But God made our bodies with many parts, and he
has put each part just where he wants it. What a strange
thing a body would be if it had only one part! Yes, there
are many parts, but only one body. The eye can never say
to the hand, "I don't need you." The head can't say to the
feet, "I don't need you."

In fact, some of the parts that seem weakest and least important are really the most necessary. And the parts we regard as less honorable are those we clothe with the greatest care. So we carefully protect from the eyes of others those parts that should not be seen, while other parts do not require this special care. So God has put the body together in such a way that extra honor and care are given to those parts that have less dignity. This makes for harmony among the members, so that all the members care for each other equally. If one part suffers, all the parts suffer with it, and if one part is honored, all the parts are glad.

Now all of you together are Christ's body, and each one of you is a separate and necessary part of it.

1 CORINTHIANS 12:12-27, NLT

Now he is far above any ruler or authority or power or leader or anything else in this world or in the world to come. And God has put all things under the authority of Christ, and he gave him this authority for the benefit of the church. And the church is his body; it is filled by Christ, who fills everything everywhere with his presence.

EPHESIANS 1:21-23, NLT

And his gifts were that some should be apostles, some prophets, some evangelists, some pastors and teachers, to equip the saints for the work of ministry, for building up

the body of Christ, until we all attain to the unity of the
faith and of the knowledge of the Son of God, to mature
manhood, to the measure of the stature of the fullness of
Christ.

EPHESIANS 4:11-13, RSV

OBSERVE THE ENEMY'S TACTICS

I was looking out the window of my house one day and saw
a simpleminded young man who lacked common sense. He
was crossing the street near the house of an immoral
woman. He was strolling down the path by her house at
twilight, as the day was fading, as the dark of night set in.
The woman approached him, dressed seductively and sly of
heart. She was the brash, rebellious type who never stays at
home. She is often seen in the streets and markets, soliciting
at every corner.

   She threw her arms around him and kissed him, and
with a brazen look she said, "I've offered my sacrifices and
just finished my vows. It's you I was looking for! I came out
to find you, and here you are! My bed is spread with colored
sheets of finest linen imported from Egypt. I've perfumed
my bed with myrrh, aloes, and cinnamon. Come, let's drink
our fill of love until morning. Let's enjoy each other's
caresses, for my husband is not home. He's away on a long
trip. He has taken a wallet full of money with him, and he
won't return until later in the month."

So she seduced him with her pretty speech. With her flattery she enticed him. He followed her at once, like an ox going to the slaughter or like a trapped stag, awaiting the arrow that would pierce its heart. He was like a bird flying into a snare, little knowing it would cost him his life.

PROVERBS 7:6-23, NLT

rules of engagement

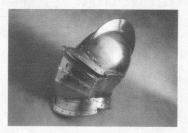

Attraction to the female body is a natural, God-given desire, so it's natural for you to find a girl's beauty tugging at your eyes for attention. You'll be tempted in many wrong ways, however, to play with these natural desires and attractions. Obviously, stripping off her clothes in the basement at the after-game party is a wrong way, but it's just as wrong to stare lustfully at her and fantasize in your mind. Neither practice is any more pure than the other.

—adapted from *Every Young Man's Battle*

LEARN TO RECOGNIZE THE SOURCE OF TEMPTATION

Then Jesus was led out into the wilderness by the Holy Spirit to be tempted there by the Devil. For forty days and forty nights he ate nothing and became very hungry. Then the Devil came and said to him, "If you are the Son of God, change these stones into loaves of bread."

MATTHEW 4:1-3, NLT

Remember, when someone wants to do wrong it is never God who is tempting him, for God never wants to do wrong and never tempts anyone else to do it. Temptation is the pull of man's own evil thoughts and wishes. These evil thoughts lead to evil actions and afterwards to the death penalty from God. So don't be misled, dear brothers.

JAMES 1:13-16, TLB

That is why, when I could bear it no longer, I sent Timothy to find out whether your faith was still strong. I was afraid that the Tempter had gotten the best of you and that all our work had been useless.

1 THESSALONIANS 3:5, NLT

But I am frightened, fearing that in some way you will be led away from your pure and simple devotion to our Lord, just as Eve was deceived by Satan in the Garden of Eden.

2 CORINTHIANS 11:3, TLB

HOW TO DEFEND AGAINST AN ENEMY ATTACK

But remember that the temptations that come into your life are no different from what others experience. And God is faithful. He will keep the temptation from becoming so strong that you can't stand up against it. When you are tempted, he will show you a way out so that you will not give in to it.

1 CORINTHIANS 10:13, NLT

If young toughs tell you, "Come and join us"—turn your back on them!

Stay far from men like that.

PROVERBS 1:10,15, TLB

The name of the LORD is a strong tower;

The righteous run to it and are safe.

PROVERBS 18:10, NKJV

Be careful—watch out for attacks from Satan, your great enemy. He prowls around like a hungry, roaring lion, looking for some victim to tear apart. Stand firm when he attacks. Trust the Lord; and remember that other Christians all around the world are going through these sufferings too.

1 PETER 5:8-9, TLB

Do not be overcome by evil, but overcome evil with good.

ROMANS 12:21, RSV

Sin is no longer your master, for you are no longer subject to the law, which enslaves you to sin. Instead, you are free by God's grace.

ROMANS 6:14, NLT

HOW TO PREPARE FOR AN ENEMY ATTACK

Watch and pray, lest you enter into temptation. The spirit indeed is willing, but the flesh is weak.

MARK 14:38, NKJV

Brethren, if a man is overtaken in any trespass, you who are spiritual should restore him in a spirit of gentleness. Look to yourself, lest you too be tempted.

GALATIANS 6:1, RSV

Be careful! Watch out for attacks from the Devil, your great enemy. He prowls around like a roaring lion, looking for some victim to devour.

1 PETER 5:8, NLT

Therefore put on the full armor of God, so that when the day of evil comes, you may be able to stand your ground, and after you have done everything, to stand.

EPHESIANS 6:13, NIV

Submit yourselves therefore to God. Resist the devil, and he will flee from you.

JAMES 4:7, KJV

A final word: Be strong with the Lord's mighty power. Put on all of God's armor so that you will be able to stand firm against all strategies and tricks of the Devil. For we are not fighting against people made of flesh and blood, but against the evil rulers and authorities of the unseen world, against those mighty powers of darkness who rule this world, and against wicked spirits in the heavenly realms.

Use every piece of God's armor to resist the enemy in the time of evil, so that after the battle you will still be standing firm. Stand your ground, putting on the sturdy belt of truth and the body armor of God's righteousness. For shoes, put on the peace that comes from the Good News, so that you will be fully prepared. In every battle you will need faith as your shield to stop the fiery arrows aimed at you by Satan. Put on salvation as your helmet, and take the sword of the Spirit, which is the word of God. Pray at all times and on every occasion in the power of the Holy Spirit. Stay alert and be persistent in your prayers for all Christians everywhere.

EPHESIANS 6:10-18, NLT

when temptation strikes

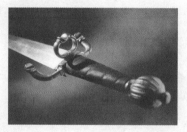

If a gang of ravenous teens were outside your home, approaching with axes and clubs, you would probably sense a threat. *Red alert! Shields up!* Just as dangerous is the woman who finds you attractive.... You have no right to indulge in sexual thoughts about her, and you have no right to return her signals!... Jesus died a bloody death on the cross to purchase you. He has all the rights here. You have none. Speak this out loudly to yourself again and again; it breaks and reins in the mustang mind.

Don't dawdle about getting your shields up!

—adapted from *Every Man's Battle*

WHEN YOU'RE ATTRACTED TO ANOTHER WOMAN

Do not lust after her beauty in your heart,
Nor let her allure you with her eyelids.
For by means of a harlot
A man is reduced to a crust of bread;
And an adulteress will prey upon his precious life.

PROVERBS 6:25-26, NKJV

Whoever commits adultery with a woman lacks
    understanding;
He who does so destroys his own soul.
Wounds and dishonor he will get,
And his reproach will not be wiped away.
For jealousy is a husband's fury;

Therefore he will not spare in the day of vengeance.
He will accept no recompense,
Nor will he be appeased though you give many
      gifts.

PROVERBS 6:32-35, NKJV

Let not your heart incline toward her ways, do not stray
into her paths.

PROVERBS 7:25, AMP

A man who loves wisdom brings joy to his father,
    but a companion of prostitutes squanders his wealth.

PROVERBS 29:3, NIV

A prudent person foresees the danger ahead and takes
precautions. The simpleton goes blindly on and suffers the
consequences.

PROVERBS 27:12, NLT

Can a man take fire to his bosom,
And his clothes not be burned?
Can one walk on hot coals,
And his feet not be seared?
So is he who goes in to his neighbor's wife;
Whoever touches her shall not be innocent.

PROVERBS 6:27-29, NKJV

WHEN A WOMAN PURSUES YOU

Wisdom will save you from the immoral woman, from the
flattery of the adulterous woman. She has abandoned her
husband and ignores the covenant she made before God.
Entering her house leads to death; it is the road to hell.
The man who visits her is doomed. He will never reach
the paths of life.

PROVERBS 2:16-19, NLT

For the lips of an immoral woman drip honey,
And her mouth is smoother than oil.

PROVERBS 5:3, NKJV

I find more bitter than death
    the woman who is a snare,
whose heart is a trap
    and whose hands are chains.
The man who pleases God will escape her,
    but the sinner she will ensnare.

ECCLESIASTES 7:26, NIV

For these commands are a lamp,
    this teaching is a light,
and the corrections of discipline
    are the way to life,
keeping you from the immoral woman,

from the smooth tongue of the wayward wife.
Do not lust in your heart after her beauty
    or let her captivate you with her eyes,
for the prostitute reduces you to a loaf of bread,
    and the adulteress preys upon your very life.

PROVERBS 6:23-26, NIV

For at the window of my house
    I have looked out through my lattice,
and I have seen among the simple,
    I have perceived among the youths,
    a young man without sense,
passing along the street near her corner,
    taking the road to her house
in the twilight, in the evening,
    at the time of night and darkness.

And lo, a woman meets him,
    dressed as a harlot, wily of heart.
She is loud and wayward,
    her feet do not stay at home;
now in the street, now in the market,
    and at every corner she lies in wait.
She seizes him and kisses him,
    and with impudent face she says to him:
"I had to offer sacrifices,
    and today I have paid my vows;

so now I have come out to meet you,

    to seek you eagerly, and I have found you.

I have decked my couch with coverings,

    colored spreads of Egyptian linen;

I have perfumed my bed with myrrh,

    aloes, and cinnamon.

Come, let us take our fill of love till morning;

    let us delight ourselves with love.

For my husband is not at home;

    he has gone on a long journey;

he took a bag of money with him;

    at full moon he will come home."

With much seductive speech she persuades

       him;

    with her smooth talk she compels him.

All at once he follows her,

    as an ox goes to the slaughter,

or as a stag is caught fast

    till an arrow pierces its entrails;

as a bird rushes into a snare;

    he does not know that it will cost him

       his life.

And now, O sons, listen to me,

    and be attentive to the words of my mouth.

Let not your heart turn aside to her ways,
    do not stray into her paths;
for many a victim has she laid low;
    yea, all her slain are a mighty host.
Her house is the way to Sheol,
    going down to the chambers of death.

PROVERBS 7:6-27, RSV

The mouth of an immoral woman is a deep pit;
He who is abhorred by the LORD will fall there.

PROVERBS 22:14, NKJV

Give me your heart, my son,
And let your eyes delight in my ways.
For a harlot is a deep pit
And an adulterous woman is a narrow well.
Surely she lurks as a robber,
And increases the faithless among men.

PROVERBS 23:26-28, NASB

Why be captivated, my son, with an immoral woman, or embrace the breasts of an adulterous woman?

PROVERBS 5:20, NLT

And I discovered more bitter than death the woman whose heart is snares and nets, whose hands are chains. One who is pleasing to God will escape from her, but the sinner will be captured by her.

ECCLESIASTES 7:26, NASB

WHEN GOD'S PLAN SEEMS TOO STRICT

It is better to spend your time at funerals than at festivals. For you are going to die, and you should think about it while there is still time.

ECCLESIASTES 7:2, NLT

Be careful! Watch out for attacks from the Devil, your great enemy. He prowls around like a roaring lion, looking for some victim to devour. Take a firm stand against him, and be strong in your faith. Remember that Christians all over the world are going through the same kind of suffering you are.

In his kindness God called you to his eternal glory by means of Jesus Christ. After you have suffered a little while, he will restore, support, and strengthen you, and he will place you on a firm foundation. All power is his forever and ever. Amen.

1 PETER 5:8-11, NLT

I saw that under the sun the race is not to the swift nor the battle to the strong…but time and chance happen to them all. For man does not know his time. Like fish which are taken in an evil net, and like birds which are caught in a snare, so the sons of men are snared at an evil time, when it suddenly falls upon them.

ECCLESIASTES 9:11,12, RSV

Man cannot abide in his pomp,
he is like the beasts that perish.

PSALM 49:12, RSV

JESUS REVEALS THE PATH OF VICTORY

When He came to the place, He said to them, "Pray that you may not enter into temptation."

LUKE 22:40, NKJV

Pray like this:
Our Father in heaven,
may your name be honored.
May your kingdom come soon.
May your Will be done here on earth,
just as it is in heaven.
Give us our food for today,
and forgive us our sins,
just as we have forgiven those who have sinned
against us.

And don't let us yield to temptation,
> but deliver us from the evil one.

MATTHEW 6:9-13, NLT

They went to a place called Gethsemane, and Jesus said to his disciples, "Sit here while I pray." He took Peter, James and John along with him, and he began to be deeply distressed and troubled. "My soul is overwhelmed with sorrow to the point of death," he said to them. "Stay here and keep watch."

Going a little farther, he fell to the ground and prayed that if possible the hour might pass from him. "Abba, Father," he said, "everything is possible for you. Take this cup from me. Yet not what I will, but what you will."

Then he returned to his disciples and found them sleeping. "Simon," he said to Peter, "are you asleep? Could you not keep watch for one hour? Watch and pray so that you will not fall into temptation. The spirit is willing, but the body is weak."

MARK 14:32-38, NIV

Then Jesus, full of the Holy Spirit, left the Jordan River, being urged by the Spirit out into the barren wastelands of Judea, where Satan tempted him for forty days. He ate nothing all that time, and was very hungry.

Satan said, "If you are God's Son, tell this stone to become a loaf of bread."

But Jesus replied, "It is written in the Scriptures, 'Other things in life are much more important than bread!'"

Then Satan took him up and revealed to him all the kingdoms of the world in a moment of time; and the devil told him, "I will give you all these splendid kingdoms and their glory—for they are mine to give to anyone I wish—if you will only get down on your knees and worship me."

Jesus replied, "We must worship God, and him alone. So it is written in the Scriptures."

Then Satan took him to Jerusalem to a high roof of the Temple and said, "If you are the Son of God, jump off! For the Scriptures say that God will send his angels to guard you and to keep you from crashing to the pavement below!"

Jesus replied, "The Scriptures also say, 'Do not put the Lord your God to a foolish test.'"

When the devil had ended all the temptations, he left Jesus for a while and went away.

Then Jesus returned to Galilee, full of the Holy Spirit's power.

LUKE 4:1-14, TLB

This High Priest of ours understands our weaknesses, for he faced all of the same temptations we do, yet he did not sin.

HEBREWS 4:15, NLT

Therefore, since the children share in flesh and blood, He Himself likewise also partook of the same, that through death He might render powerless him who had the power of death, that is, the devil, and might free those who through fear of death were subject to slavery all their lives. For assuredly He does not give help to angels, but He gives help to the descendant of Abraham. Therefore, He had to be made like His brethren in all things, so that He might become a merciful and faithful high priest in things pertaining to God, to make propitiation for the sins of the people. For since He Himself was tempted in that which He has suffered, He is able to come to the aid of those who are tempted.

HEBREWS 2:14-18, NASB

pride sets you up for a fall, so don't stop short

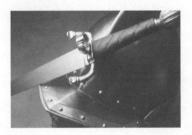

Knowing that God's standard is the standard of true life, Josiah rose up and tore down *everything* that was in opposition to God.... And what about you? Now that you've heard about God's standard of sexual purity, are you willing, in the spirit of Josiah, to make a covenant to hold to that standard with all your heart and soul? Will you tear down every sexual thing that stands in opposition to God?

Can you see that you've been living the mixed standards of mere excellence? Stopping short but still looking Christian enough?

Or have you aimed for obedience and perfection, where you're truly called to go?

—Every Man's Battle

BROKENNESS COMES WITH PRIDE

Pride goes before destruction,
    and a haughty spirit before a fall.

PROVERBS 16:18, RSV

Haughtiness goes before destruction; humility precedes honor.

PROVERBS 18:12, NLT

For many walk, of whom I have told you often, and now tell you even weeping, that they are the enemies of the

cross of Christ: whose end is destruction, whose god is
their belly, and whose glory is in their shame—who set
their mind on earthly things.

PHILIPPIANS 3:18, NKJV

Haughty eyes and a proud heart,
    the lamp of the wicked, are sin.

PROVERBS 21:4, RSV

Enter through the narrow gate; for wide is the gate
and spacious and broad is the way that leads away
to destruction, and many are those who are entering
through it.

MATTHEW 7:13, AMP

But there were also false prophets among the people, just
as there will be false teachers among you. They will secretly
introduce destructive heresies, even denying the sovereign
Lord who bought them—bringing swift destruction on
themselves.

2 PETER 2:1, NIV

Though you already know all this, I want to remind you
that the Lord delivered his people out of Egypt, but later
destroyed those who did not believe.

JUDE 5, NIV

WHAT PRIDE WILL DO TO YOU

But when [Uzziah] became strong, his heart was so proud that he acted corruptly, and he was unfaithful to the LORD his God.

2 CHRONICLES 26:16, NASB

The LORD despises pride; be assured that the proud will be punished.

PROVERBS 16:5, NLT

The Lord hates the stubborn but delights in those who are good. You can be very sure that the evil man will not go unpunished forever. And you can also be very sure that God will rescue the children of the godly.

PROVERBS 11:20-21, TLB

Better it is to be of an humble spirit with the lowly, than to divide the spoil with the proud.

PROVERBS 16:19, KJV

The LORD mocks at mockers, but he shows favor to the humble.

PROVERBS 3:34, NLT

Pride goes before destruction.

PROVERBS 16:18, NIV

DISCOVER THE POWER OF HUMILITY

By humility and the fear of the LORD are riches, and honour, and life.

PROVERBS 22:4, KJV

When pride comes, then comes dishonor,
But with the humble is wisdom.

PROVERBS 11:2, NASB

Heaven is my throne and the earth is my footstool.... My hand has made both earth and skies, and they are mine. Yet I will look with pity on the man who has a humble and a contrite heart, who trembles at my word.

ISAIAH 66:1,2, TLB

A man's pride will bring him low,
But a humble spirit will obtain honor.

PROVERBS 29:23, NASB

For whoever exalts himself will be humbled, and he who humbles himself will be exalted.

LUKE 14:11, NKJV

But the humble will inherit the land,
And will delight themselves in abundant prosperity.

PSALM 37:11, NASB

Fear of the LORD teaches a person to be wise; humility precedes honor.

PROVERBS 15:33, NLT

Humble yourselves in the sight of the Lord, and he shall lift you up.

JAMES 4:10, KJV

when you've fallen into sin

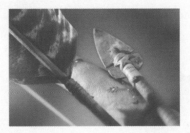

FACING THE GRAVITY OF YOUR SIN

O my God, I am too ashamed and disgraced to lift up my
face to you, my God, because our sins are higher than our
heads and our guilt has reached to the heavens.

EZRA 9:6, NIV

O loving and kind God, have mercy. Have pity upon me
and take away the awful stain of my transgressions. Oh,
wash me, cleanse me from this guilt. Let me be pure again.
For I admit my shameful deed—it haunts me day and
night. It is against you and you alone I sinned and did this
terrible thing. You saw it all, and your sentence against me
is just. But I was born a sinner, yes, from the moment my
mother conceived me. You deserve honesty from the heart;
yes, utter sincerity and truthfulness. Oh, give me this
wisdom.

Sprinkle me with the cleansing blood and I shall be
clean again. Wash me and I shall be whiter than snow. And
after you have punished me, give me back my joy again.
Don't keep looking at my sins—erase them from your
sight. Create in me a new, clean heart, O God, filled with
clean thoughts and right desires. Don't toss me aside, ban-
ished forever from your presence. Don't take your Holy
Spirit from me. Restore to me again the joy of your salvation, and make me willing to obey you.

PSALM 51:1-12, TLB

If we say that we have no sin, we are deceiving ourselves, and the truth is not in us. If we confess our sins, He is faithful and righteous to forgive us our sins and to cleanse us from all unrighteousness. If we say that we have not sinned, we make Him a liar, and His word is not in us.

1 JOHN 1:8-10, NASB

God doesn't listen to the prayers of men who flout the law.

PROVERBS 28:9, TLB

FORGIVENESS IS JUST A PRAYER AWAY

If we confess our sins, he is faithful and just to forgive us our sins, and to cleanse us from all unrighteousness.

1 JOHN 1:9, KJV

Answer me when I call, O God of my righteousness!
You have relieved me in my distress;
Be gracious to me and hear my prayer.

PSALM 4:1, NASB

For this is what the high and lofty One says—
    he who lives forever, whose name is holy:
"I live in a high and holy place,
    but also with him who is contrite and lowly in spirit,
to revive the spirit of the lowly
    and to revive the heart of the contrite.

"I will not accuse forever,
>   nor will I always be angry,
for then the spirit of man would grow faint before me—
>   the breath of man that I have created."

ISAIAH 57:15-16, NIV

Come, let us return to the LORD;
>   for he has torn, that he may heal us;
>   he has stricken, and he will bind us up.
After two days he will revive us;
>   on the third day he will raise us up,
>   that we may live before him.
Let us know, let us press on to know the LORD;
>   his going forth is sure as the dawn;
he will come to us as the showers,
>   as the spring rains that water the earth.

HOSEA 6:1-3, RSV

Finally, I confessed all my sins to you
>   and stopped trying to hide them.
I said to myself, "I will confess my rebellion to the LORD."

PSALM 32:5, NLT

A man who refuses to admit his mistakes can never be successful. But if he confesses and forsakes them, he gets another chance.

PROVERBS 28:13, TLB

But He, being full of compassion, forgave their iniquity,
And did not destroy them.
Yes, many a time He turned His anger away,
And did not stir up all His wrath.

PSALM 78:38, NKJV

TURN YOUR BACK ON SIN

"The time has come," he said. "The kingdom of God is
near. Repent and believe the good news!"

MARK 1:15, NIV

Repent therefore, and turn again, that your sins may be
blotted out, that times of refreshing may come from the
presence of the Lord.

ACTS 3:19, RSV

"Don't tear your clothing in your grief; instead, tear your
hearts." Return to the LORD your God, for he is gracious
and merciful. He is not easily angered. He is filled with
kindness and is eager not to punish you.

JOEL 2:13, NLT

The Lord is not slow about His promise, as some count
slowness, but is patient toward you, not wishing for any to
perish but for all to come to repentance.

2 PETER 3:9, NASB

Another reason for right living is that you know how late it is; time is running out. Wake up, for the coming of our salvation is nearer now than when we first believed.

ROMANS 13:11, NLT

Or do you think lightly of the riches of His kindness and tolerance and patience, not knowing that the kindness of God leads you to repentance?

ROMANS 2:4, NASB

He is so rich in kindness that he purchased our freedom through the blood of his Son, and our sins are forgiven.

EPHESIANS 1:7, NLT

I pray that your hearts will be flooded with light so that you can understand the wonderful future he has promised to those he called. I want you to realize what a rich and glorious inheritance he has given to his people.

EPHESIANS 1:18, NLT

For I [Paul] am afraid that when I come to visit you I won't like what I find.… And I will have to grieve because many of you who sinned earlier have not repented of your impurity, sexual immorality, and eagerness for lustful pleasure.

2 CORINTHIANS 12:20,21, NLT

WHEN YOU THINK YOU'RE BEYOND HELP

Let, I pray thee, thy merciful kindness be for my comfort, according to thy word unto thy servant.

PSALM 119:76, KJV

For you were straying like sheep, but have now returned to the Shepherd and Guardian of your souls.

1 PETER 2:25, RSV

I will search for my lost ones who strayed away, and I will bring them safely home again. I will bind up the injured and strengthen the weak. But I will destroy those who are fat and powerful. I will feed them, yes—feed them justice!

EZEKIEL 34:16, NLT

Once you were alienated from God and were enemies in your minds because of your evil behavior. But now he has reconciled you by Christ's physical body through death to present you holy in his sight, without blemish and free from accusation.

COLOSSIANS 1:21-22, NIV

Rejoice always, pray constantly, give thanks in all circumstances; for this is the will of God in Christ Jesus for you.

1 THESSALONIANS 5:16-18, RSV

WHEN YOU NEED A REMINDER THAT GOD ANSWERS PRAYER

I cried out to the LORD in my great trouble, and he
answered me. I called to you from the world of the dead,
and LORD, you heard me!

JONAH 2:2, NLT

But he who endures to the end will be saved.

MATTHEW 24:13, AMP

I love the LORD because he hears
    and answers my prayers.
Because he bends down and listens,
    I will pray as long as I have breath!

PSALM 116:1-2, NLT

Depart from me, all you who do iniquity,
For the LORD has heard the voice of my weeping.

PSALM 6:8, NASB

But certainly God has heard me;
He has attended to the voice of my prayer.

PSALM 66:19, NKJV

Why am I praying like this? Because I know you will
answer me, O God! Yes, listen as I pray.

PSALM 17:6, TLB

The eyes of the LORD are toward the righteous,
And His ears are open to their cry.

PSALM 34:15, NASB

He will fulfill the desire of those who fear Him;
He will also hear their cry and will save them.

PSALM 145:19, NASB

Well, God doesn't listen to evil men, but he has open ears
to those who worship him and do his will.

JOHN 9:31, TLB

Incline Your ear to me, rescue me quickly;
Be to me a rock of strength,
A stronghold to save me.

PSALM 31:2, NASB

Blessed be God,
Who has not turned away my prayer
Nor His lovingkindness from me.

PSALM 66:20, NASB

God wants the best for you

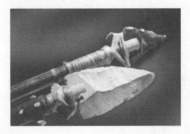

WHEN YOU THINK GOD IS ANGRY WITH YOU

He passed in front of Moses and said, "I am the LORD, I am the LORD, the merciful and gracious God. I am slow to anger and rich in unfailing love and faithfulness."

EXODUS 34:6, NLT

The LORD is slow to anger and abundant in lovingkindness, forgiving iniquity and transgression.

NUMBERS 14:18, NASB

For the LORD your God is a compassionate God; He will not fail you nor destroy you nor forget the covenant with your fathers which He swore to them.

DEUTERONOMY 4:31, NASB

For His anger is but for a moment,
His favor is for life;
Weeping may endure for a night,
But joy comes in the morning.

PSALM 30:5, NKJV

The LORD is compassionate and gracious,
Slow to anger and abounding in lovingkindness.
He will not always strive with us,
Nor will He keep His anger forever.
He has not dealt with us according to our sins,

Nor rewarded us according to our iniquities.
For as high as the heavens are above the earth,
So great is His lovingkindness toward those who
     fear Him.
As far as the east is from the west,
So far has He removed our transgressions from us.
Just as a father has compassion on his children,
So the LORD has compassion on those who fear Him.
For He Himself knows our frame;
He is mindful that we are but dust.

PSALM 103:8-14, NASB

But You, O LORD, are a God merciful and gracious,
Slow to anger and abundant in lovingkindness and
     truth.

PSALM 86:15, NASB

They refused to listen,
And did not remember Your wondrous deeds which You
     had performed among them;
So they became stubborn and appointed a leader to return
     to their slavery in Egypt.
But You are a God of forgiveness,
Gracious and compassionate,
Slow to anger and abounding in lovingkindness;
And You did not forsake them.

NEHEMIAH 9:17, NASB

For I [know] you [are] a gracious God, merciful, slow to
get angry, and full of kindness; I [know] how easily you
could cancel your plans for destroying these people.

JONAH 4:2, TLB

WHEN YOU NEED TO BE REMINDED OF GOD'S HOPE

O God, we have heard it with our own ears—
     our ancestors have told us
of all you did in other days,
     in days long ago…
you crushed their enemies,
     setting our ancestors free.…
It was by your mighty power that they succeeded;
     it was because you favored them and smiled on them.

PSALM 44:1,2,3, NLT

You threw me into the ocean depths, and I sank down to the
heart of the sea. I was buried beneath your wild and stormy
waves. Then I said, "O LORD, you have driven me from your
presence. How will I ever again see your holy Temple?"

I sank beneath the waves, and death was very near.
The waters closed in around me, and seaweed wrapped
itself around my head. I sank down to the very roots of the
mountains. I was locked out of life and imprisoned in the
land of the dead. But you, O LORD my God, have
snatched me from the yawning jaws of death!

When I had lost all hope, I turned my thoughts once more to the LORD.

JONAH 2:3-7, NLT

And when God saw that they had put a stop to their evil ways, he abandoned his plan to destroy them, and didn't carry it through.

JONAH 3:10, TLB

And you will be hated by all men for My name's sake. But he who endures to the end shall be saved.

MARK 13:13, NKJV

Many are the woes of the wicked,
    but the LORD's unfailing love
    surrounds the man who trusts in him.

PSALM 32:10, NIV

"No weapon that is formed against you will prosper.…
This is the heritage of the servants of the LORD,
And their vindication is from Me," declares the LORD.

ISAIAH 54:17, NASB

For it is by grace you have been saved, through faith—and this not from yourselves, it is the gift of God—not by works, so that no one can boast.

EPHESIANS 2:8-9, NIV

Now faith is the assurance of things hoped for, the conviction of things not seen.

HEBREWS 11:1, RSV

And we desire each one of you to show the same earnestness in realizing the full assurance of hope until the end, so that you may not be sluggish, but imitators of those who through faith and patience inherit the promises.

HEBREWS 6:11-12, RSV

We have this as a sure and steadfast anchor of the soul, a hope...

HEBREWS 6:19, RSV

Now we are the sons of God, and it doth not yet appear what we shall be: but we know that, when he shall appear, we shall be like him; for we shall see him as he is. And every man that hath this hope in him purifieth himself, even as he is pure.

1 JOHN 3:2,3, KJV

For God has not destined us for wrath, but to obtain salvation through our Lord Jesus Christ, who died for us so that whether we wake or sleep we might live with him. Therefore encourage one another and build one another up, just as you are doing.

1 THESSALONIANS 5:9-11, RSV

WHEN YOU NEED TO BE REMINDED THAT GOD HAS A PLAN FOR YOU

Say to the righteous that it will go well with them,
For they will eat the fruit of their actions.

ISAIAH 3:10, NASB

Although a sinner does evil a hundred times and may lengthen his life, still I know that it will be well for those who fear God, who fear Him openly.

ECCLESIASTES 8:12, NASB

Now it shall be, if you diligently obey the LORD your God, being careful to do all His commandments…the LORD your God will set you high above all the nations of the earth.

DEUTERONOMY 28:1, NASB

Take the old prophets as your mentors. They put up with anything, went through everything, and never once quit, all the time honoring God. What a gift life is to those who stay the course! You've heard, of course, of Job's staying power, and you know how God brought it all together for him at the end. That's because God cares, cares right down to the last detail.

JAMES 5:11, MSG

He saved us, not because of righteous things we had done, but because of his mercy. He saved us through the washing of rebirth and renewal by the Holy Spirit.

TITUS 3:5, NIV

All these blessings shall come upon you and overtake you, if you obey the voice of the LORD your God. Blessed shall you be in the city, and blessed shall you be in the field. Blessed shall be the fruit of your body, and the fruit of your ground, and the fruit of your beasts, the increase of your cattle, and the young of your flock. Blessed shall be your basket and your kneading-trough. Blessed shall you be when you come in, and blessed shall you be when you go out.

The LORD will cause your enemies who rise up against you to be defeated before you; they shall come out against you one way, and flee before you seven ways. The LORD will command the blessing upon you in your barns, and in all that you undertake; and he will bless you in the land which the LORD your God gives you. The LORD will establish you as a people holy to himself, as he has sworn to you, if you keep the commandments of the LORD your God, and walk in his ways. And all the peoples of the earth shall see that you are called by the name of the LORD; and they shall be afraid of you. And the LORD will make you abound in prosperity, in the fruit of your body, and in the fruit of your cattle, and in the fruit of your ground, within the land which the LORD swore to your fathers to give you. The LORD will open to you his good treasury the heavens, to give the rain of your land in its season and to bless all the work of your hands; and you shall lend to many nations.

DEUTERONOMY 28:2-12, RSV

you've been called to fight

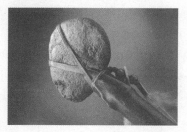

Our heavenly Father exhorts us to be men. He wants us to be like Him. When He calls us to "be perfect as your Father in heaven is perfect," He's asking us to rise above our natural tendencies to impure eyes, fanciful minds, and wandering hearts. While understanding that His standard of purity doesn't come naturally to us, He still calls us to rise up, by the power of His indwelling presence, to get the job done.

Before an important battle for the army he commanded, Joab said to the troops of Israel, "Be of good courage, and let us play the men for our people" (2 Samuel 10:12, KJV). In short, he was saying, "We know God's plan for us. Let's rise up as men, and set our hearts and minds to get it done!"

In the realm of sexual integrity, God wants *you* to rise up and get it done.

—adapted from *Every Man's Battle*

THE COMMAND TO BREAK FREE

We have power through the Lord to overcome every level of sexual immorality, but if we don't utilize that power, we'll never break free of the habit.

—*Every Man's Battle*

Dearest friends, when I [Paul] was there with you, you were always so careful to follow my instructions. And now that I am away you must be even more careful to do the good things that result from being saved, obeying God with deep reverence, shrinking back from all that might displease him. For God is at work within you, helping you want to obey him, and…helping you do what he wants.

PHILIPPIANS 2:12-13, TLB

Since you have been raised to new life with Christ, set your sights on the realities of heaven, where Christ sits at God's right hand in the place of honor and power.

COLOSSIANS 3:1, NLT

I will give you a new heart with new and right desires, and I will put a new spirit in you. I will take out your stony heart of sin and give you a new, obedient heart. And I will put my Spirit in you so you will obey my laws and do whatever I command.

EZEKIEL 36:26-27, NLT

No one who is born of God will continue to sin, because God's seed remains in him; he cannot go on sinning, because he has been born of God.

1 JOHN 3:9, NIV

THE COMMAND TO CHOOSE MANHOOD

When it comes down to it, God's definition of real manhood is pretty simple: It means hearing His Word and *doing it*. That's God's *only* definition of manhood—a doer of the Word. And God's definition of a sissy is someone who hears the Word of God and *doesn't* do it. When you make a covenant to be sexually pure, to rise above your natural male tendencies, you make a choice for true manhood.

—adapted from *Every Man's Battle*

I am speaking in human terms because of the weakness of your flesh. For just as you presented your members as slaves to impurity and to lawlessness, resulting in further lawlessness, so now present your members as slaves to righteousness, resulting in sanctification.

ROMANS 6:19, NASB

Since everything around us is going to melt away, what holy, godly lives you should be living!

2 PETER 3:11, NLT

Therefore do not let sin reign in your mortal body, that you should obey it in its lusts.

ROMANS 6:12, NKJV

THE COMMAND TO COURAGEOUSLY TAKE HOLD OF GOD'S PROVISION

It's like the situation facing Joshua and the people of Israel as they prepared to cross the Jordan River and possess the Promised Land. What did God say to Joshua?

"Have I not commanded you? Be strong and courageous! Do not be terrified; do not be discouraged, *for the LORD your God will be with you wherever you go*" (Joshua 1:9, [NIV, emphasis added]).

He'd given the Israelites all they needed. They merely had to cross the river.

Regarding sexual purity, God knows the provision He's made for us. We aren't short on power or authority, but what we lack is *urgency.* We must choose to be strong and courageous to walk into purity. In the millisecond it takes to make that choice, the Holy Spirit will start guiding you and walking through the struggle with you.

—Every Man's Battle

Be strong and show yourself a man; keep the charge of the Lord your God, walk in His ways, keep His statutes, His commandments, His precepts, and His testimonies…that you may do wisely and prosper in all that you do and wherever you turn.

1 KINGS 2:2-3, AMP

Be on your guard; stand firm in the faith; be men of courage; be strong.

1 CORINTHIANS 16:13, NIV

Finally, my brethren, be strong in the Lord, and in the power of his might.

EPHESIANS 6:10, KJV

THE COMMAND TO ABSTAIN

Abstain from all appearance of evil.

1 Thessalonians 5:22, kjv

God wants you to be holy, so you should keep clear of all sexual sin. Then each of you will control your body and live in holiness and honor—not in lustful passion as the pagans do, in their ignorance of God and his ways.

1 Thessalonians 4:3-5, nlt

Beloved, I urge you as aliens and strangers to abstain from fleshly lusts which wage war against the soul.

1 Peter 2:11, nasb

THE COMMAND TO PURIFY YOURSELF

Since we have these promises, dear friends, let us purify ourselves from everything that contaminates body and spirit, perfecting holiness out of reverence for God.

2 Corinthians 7:1, niv

Wash and make yourselves clean.
Take your evil deeds
out of my sight!
Stop doing wrong.

Isaiah 1:16, niv

But in a great house there are not only vessels of gold and silver, but also of wood and clay, some for honor and some for dishonor.

Therefore if anyone cleanses himself from the latter, he will be a vessel for honor, sanctified and useful for the Master, prepared for every good work.

2 TIMOTHY 2:20-21, NKJV

Draw near to God and He will draw near to you. Cleanse your hands, you sinners; and purify your hearts.

JAMES 4:8, NASB

THE COMMAND TO LIVE IN A WAY THAT PLEASES GOD

Finally, dear brothers and sisters, we urge you in the name of the Lord Jesus to live in a way that pleases God, as we have taught you. You are doing this already, and we encourage you to do so more and more.

1 THESSALONIANS 4:1, NLT

As obedient children, do not conform to the evil desires you had when you lived in ignorance. But just as he who called you is holy, so be holy in all you do.

1 PETER 1:14-15, NIV

And you know that we treated each of you as a father treats his own children. We pleaded with you, encouraged you, and urged you to live your lives in a way that God would consider worthy. For he called you into his Kingdom to share his glory.

1 Thessalonians 2:11-12, nlt

As a prisoner for the Lord, then, I urge you to live a life worthy of the calling you have received.

Ephesians 4:1, niv

THE COMMAND TO GROW IN KNOWLEDGE

But grow in the grace and knowledge of our Lord and Savior Jesus Christ. To him be the glory both now and to the day of eternity. Amen.

2 Peter 3:18, rsv

"But let him who boasts boast of this, that he understands and knows Me, that I am the LORD who exercises lovingkindness, justice and righteousness on earth; for I delight in these things," declares the LORD.

Jeremiah 9:24, nasb

And if you call out for insight
and cry aloud for understanding,
and if you look for it as for silver
and search for it as for hidden treasure,

then you will understand the fear of the LORD
   and find the knowledge of God.

PROVERBS 2:3-5, NIV

Happy (blessed, fortunate, enviable) is the man who finds
skillful and godly Wisdom, and the man who gets understanding [drawing it forth from God's Word and life's
experiences].

PROVERBS 3:13, AMP

Get wisdom, get understanding: forget it not; neither
decline from the words of my mouth.

PROVERBS 4:5, KJV

But also for this very reason, giving all diligence, add to
your faith virtue, to virtue knowledge.

2 PETER 1:5, NKJV

And you will know the truth, and the truth will set
you free.

JOHN 8:32, NLT

THE COMMAND TO FLEE

Run from all these evil things, and work instead at what is
right and good, learning to trust him and love others and
to be patient and gentle. Fight on for God. Hold tightly to

the eternal life that God has given you and that you have confessed with such a ringing confession before many witnesses.

1 TIMOTHY 6:11-12, TLB

Flee from sexual immorality. All other sins a man commits are outside his body, but he who sins sexually sins against his own body.

1 CORINTHIANS 6:18, NIV

Now flee from youthful lusts and pursue righteousness, faith, love and peace, with those who call on the Lord from a pure heart.

2 TIMOTHY 2:22, NASB

Therefore, my dear friends, flee from idolatry.

1 CORINTHIANS 10:14, NIV

THE COMMAND TO LIVE AS CHILDREN OF THE LIGHT

The night is nearly over; the day is almost here. So let us put aside the deeds of darkness and put on the armor of light. Let us behave decently, as in the daytime, not in orgies and drunkenness, not in sexual immorality and debauchery, not in dissension and jealousy. Rather, clothe yourselves with the Lord Jesus Christ, and do not think about how to gratify the desires of the sinful nature.

ROMANS 13:12-14, NIV

For though your hearts were once full of darkness, now you are full of light from the Lord, and your behavior should show it! For this light within you produces only what is good and right and true.

Try to find out what is pleasing to the Lord. Take no part in the worthless deeds of evil and darkness; instead, rebuke and expose them.

EPHESIANS 5:8-11, NLT

For you are all children of the light and of the day; we don't belong to darkness and night. So be on your guard, not asleep like the others. Stay alert and be sober.

1 THESSALONIANS 5:5-6, NLT

THE COMMAND TO PUT ON THE NEW SELF

You were taught, with regard to your former way of life, to put off your old self, which is being corrupted by its deceitful desires; to be made new in the attitude of your minds; and to put on the new self, created to be like God in true righteousness and holiness.

EPHESIANS 4:22-24, NIV

Therefore, if anyone is in Christ, he is a new creation; the old has gone, the new has come!

2 CORINTHIANS 5:17, NIV

Our old sinful selves were crucified with Christ so that sin might lose its power in our lives. We are no longer slaves to sin.

ROMANS 6:6, NLT

THE COMMAND TO LIVE DIFFERENTLY FROM THE WORLD

Let me say this, then, speaking for the Lord: Live no longer as the unsaved do, for they are blinded and confused. Their closed hearts are full of darkness; they are far away from the life of God because they have shut their minds against him, and they cannot understand his ways. They don't care anymore about right and wrong and have given themselves over to impure ways. They stop at nothing, being driven by their evil minds and reckless lusts.

EPHESIANS 4:17-19, TLB

For you have spent enough time in the past doing what the pagans choose to do—living in debauchery, lust, drunkenness, orgies, carousing and detestable idolatry. They think it strange that you do not plunge with them into the same flood of dissipation, and they heap abuse on

you. But they will have to give account to him who is
ready to judge the living and the dead.

1 PETER 4:3-5, NIV

If anyone loves the world, the love of the Father is not in
him. For everything in the world—the cravings of sinful
man, the lust of his eyes and the boasting of what he has
and does—comes not from the Father but from the world.
The world and its desires pass away, but the man who does
the will of God lives forever.

1 JOHN 2:15-17, NIV

THE COMMAND TO GUARD YOUR HEART AND TO EXHIBIT SELF-CONTROL

Above all else, guard your heart, for it affects everything
you do.

PROVERBS 4:23, NLT

Set your affection on things above, not on things on the
earth.

COLOSSIANS 3:2, KJV

But the fruit of the Spirit is love, joy, peace, patience, kindness, goodness, faithfulness, gentleness, self-control;
against such there is no law.

GALATIANS 5:22-23, RSV

A man without self-control
    is like a city broken into and left without walls.

PROVERBS 25:28, RSV

For as you know him better, he will give you, through his
great power, everything you need for living a truly good
life: he even shares his own glory and his own goodness
with us! And by that same mighty power he has given us
all the other rich and wonderful blessings he promised; for
instance, the promise to save us from the lust and rotten-
ness all around us, and to give us his own character.

    But to obtain these gifts, you need more than faith;
you must also work hard to be good, and even that is not
enough. For then you must learn to know God better and
discover what he wants you to do. Next, learn to put aside
your own desires so that you will become patient and
godly, gladly letting God have his way with you. This will
make possible the next step, which is for you to enjoy
other people and to like them, and finally you will grow to
love them deeply. The more you go on in this way, the
more you will grow strong spiritually and become fruitful
and useful to our Lord Jesus Christ.

2 PETER 1:3-8, TLB

Be self-controlled and alert. Your enemy the devil prowls
around like a roaring lion looking for someone to devour.

Resist him, standing firm in the faith, because you know
that your brothers throughout the world are undergoing
the same kind of sufferings.

And the God of all grace, who called you to his eternal
glory in Christ, after you have suffered a little while, will
himself restore you and make you strong, firm and steadfast. To him be the power for ever and ever. Amen.

1 PETER 5:8-11, NIV

The end of all things is near. Therefore be clear minded
and self-controlled so that you can pray.

1 PETER 4:7, NIV

Now a bishop (superintendent, overseer) must give
no grounds for accusation but must be above reproach,
the husband of one wife, circumspect and temperate
and self-controlled; [he must be] sensible and well
behaved and dignified and lead an orderly (disciplined)
life.

1 TIMOTHY 3:2, AMP

For God did not give us a spirit of timidity (of cowardice,
of craven and cringing and fawning fear), but [He has
given us a spirit] of power and of love and of calm and
well-balanced mind and discipline and self-control.

2 TIMOTHY 1:7, AMP

Therefore, prepare your minds for action; be self-
controlled; set your hope fully on the grace to be given
you when Jesus Christ is revealed.

1 PETER 1:13, NIV

THE COMMAND TO BECOME BLAMELESS

Holiness is not some nebulous thing. It's a series of right choices.
You needn't wait for some holy cloud to form around you. You'll be
holy when you choose not to sin. You're already free from the
power of sexual immorality; you are not yet free from the *habit* of
sexual immorality, until you choose to be—until you say, "That's
enough! I'm choosing to live purely!"

—*Every Man's Battle*

Do everything without complaining or arguing, so that
you may become blameless and pure, children of God
without fault in a crooked and depraved generation, in
which you shine like stars in the universe as you hold out
the word of life.

PHILIPPIANS 2:14-16, NIV

So then, dear friends, since you are looking forward to
this, make every effort to be found spotless, blameless and
at peace with him.

2 PETER 3:14, NIV

For all his laws are constantly before me;
> I have never abandoned his principles.
I am blameless before God;
> I have kept myself from sin.
The LORD rewarded me for doing right,
> because of the innocence of my hands in his sight.
To the faithful you show yourself faithful;
> to those with integrity you show integrity.

PSALM 18:22-25, NLT

Righteousness keeps him whose way is blameless.

PROVERBS 13:6, NKJV

I will be careful to lead a blameless life—
> when will you come to me?
I will walk in my house
> with blameless heart.

PSALM 101:2, NIV

He holds victory in store for the upright,
> he is a shield to those whose walk is blameless.

PROVERBS 2:7, NIV

And this I pray, that your love may abound still more
and more in real knowledge and all discernment, so
that you may approve the things that are excellent, in

order to be sincere and blameless until the day of Christ;
having been filled with the fruit of righteousness which
comes through Jesus Christ, to the glory and praise of God.

PHILIPPIANS 1:9-11, NASB

In view of this, I also do my best to maintain always a
blameless conscience both before God and before men.

ACTS 24:16, NASB

THE COMMAND TO OBEY

At a single moment, salvation gave us a new life and a new desire
to be sexually pure for the first time. But this new desire alone will
not bring full intimacy with Christ. We must say yes to this new
desire and refuse to ignore it. We must choose oneness and intimacy with Christ. We must choose sexual purity.

—*Every Young Man's Battle*

Therefore whoever hears these sayings of Mine, and does
them, I will liken him to a wise man who built his house
on the rock.

MATTHEW 7:24, NKJV

But if you do not obey the LORD, and if you rebel against
his commands, his hand will be against you, as it was
against your fathers.

1 SAMUEL 12:15, NIV

In God's kingdom, Old Testament or New Testament, choosing obedience has always been central to intimacy with God. Trouble is, we aren't in search of obedience. We're in search of mere excellence, and His command is *not* enough. We push back, responding, "*Why should I eliminate every hint? That's too hard!*"

We have countless churches filled with countless men encumbered by sexual sin, weakened by low-grade sexual fevers—men happy enough to go to Promise Keepers but too sickly to *be* promise keepers.

A spiritual battle for purity is going on in every heart and soul. The costs are real. Obedience is hard, requiring humility and meekness, very rare elements indeed.

—adapted from *Every Man's Battle*

Don't you realize that whatever you choose to obey
becomes your master? You can choose sin, which leads to
death, or you can choose to obey God and receive his
approval.

ROMANS 6:16, NLT

Does the Lord delight in burnt offerings and sacrifices
    as much as in obeying the voice of the LORD?
To obey is better than sacrifice,
    and to heed is better than the fat of rams.
For rebellion is like the sin of divination,
    and arrogance like the evil of idolatry.

1 SAMUEL 15:22–23, NIV

This is love for God: to obey his commands. And his commands are not burdensome, for everyone born of God overcomes the world.

1 JOHN 5:3-4, NIV

the basics of planning for battle

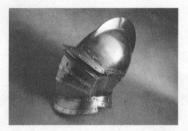

Our objective in the war against lust is *to build three perimeters of defense* into our lives: (1) With our eyes; (2) in our minds; and (3) in our hearts.

Think of the first perimeter (your eyes) as your outermost defense. Just as Job made a covenant with his eyes not to look lustfully at a girl, you can do the same by training your eyes to *bounce* from objects of lust.

With the second perimeter (your mind), you don't so much block out the objects of lust, but you *evaluate* and *capture* them. A key verse is 2 Corinthians 10:5: "We take captive every thought to make it obedient to Christ" (NIV).

Your third objective is to build your innermost defense perimeter—in your heart. This perimeter is built by strengthening your affections for your wife and your commitment to the promises and debts you owe her. Your marriage can die from within if you neglect your promise to love, honor, and cherish your wife. *Honoring* and *cherishing* are your key actions in establishing this defense perimeter.

So there's your battle plan. You set up defense perimeters and choose not to sin. You'll have freedom from sexual impurity as soon as those defense perimeters are in place.

—adapted from *Every Man's Battle*

WISE WARRIORS ALWAYS HAVE A PLAN

A wise man is mightier than a strong man, and a man of knowledge is more powerful than a strong man. So don't go to war without wise guidance; victory depends on having many counselors.

PROVERBS 24:5-6, NLT

Prepare plans by consultation,
And make war by wise guidance.

PROVERBS 20:18, NASB

I am warning you ahead of time, dear friends, so that you can watch out and not be carried away by the errors of these wicked people. I don't want you to lose your own secure footing.

2 PETER 3:17, NLT

OUR PLANS NEED TO BE IN SYNC WITH GOD'S

Human plans, no matter how wise or well advised, cannot stand against the LORD.

PROVERBS 21:30, NLT

The one who despises the word will be in debt to it,
But the one who fears the commandment will be rewarded.

PROVERBS 13:13, NASB

There are many devices in a man's heart; nevertheless the counsel of the LORD, that shall stand.

PROVERBS 19:21, KJV

No one serving as a soldier gets involved in civilian affairs—he wants to please his commanding officer.

2 TIMOTHY 2:4, NIV

GOD HAS BIG PLANS FOR THOSE WHO FOLLOW HIS LEAD

"For I know the plans I have for you," declares the LORD, "plans to prosper you and not to harm you, plans to give you hope and a future."

JEREMIAH 29:11, NIV

I will let every one who conquers sit beside me on my throne, just as I took my place with my Father on his throne when I had conquered.

REVELATION 3:21, TLB

To him who overcomes and does my will to the end, I will give authority over the nations.

REVELATION 2:26, NIV

I have told you all this so that you may have peace in me. Here on earth you will have many trials and sorrows. But take heart, because I have overcome the world.

JOHN 16:33, NLT

a battle plan for the eyes and mind

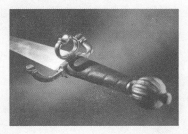

It's critical to recognize visual sexual impurity as foreplay. If viewing sensual things merely provides a flutter of appreciation for a woman's beauty, it would be no different than viewing the awesome power of a thunderstorm racing over the Iowa cornfields. No sin. No problem.

But if it *is* foreplay, and if you're getting sexual gratification from images of women, you are defiling the marriage bed.

The problem is that your eyes have always bounced toward the sexual, and you've made no attempt to end this habit. To combat it, you need to build a reflex action by training your eyes to immediately bounce away from the sexual, like the jerk of your hand away from a hot stove.

—**adapted from *Every Man's Battle***

FIX YOUR EYES ON THE STRAIGHT AND NARROW

I will set before my eyes
　　no vile thing.

PSALM 101:3, NIV

Turn away my eyes from looking at worthless things,
And revive me in Your way.

PSALM 119:37, NKJV

I will tell you who can live here: All who are honest and
fair,…who shut their eyes to all enticement to do wrong.

ISAIAH 33:15, TLB

Look straight ahead, and fix your eyes on what lies before
you. Mark out a straight path for your feet; then stick to
the path and stay safe. Don't get sidetracked; keep your
feet from following evil.

PROVERBS 4:25-27, NLT

If your right eye causes you to sin, gouge it out and throw
it away. It is better for you to lose one part of your body
than for your whole body to be thrown into hell.

MATTHEW 5:29, NIV

DON'T UNDERESTIMATE THE POWER OF LUST

If you want freedom from sexual sin, you must put the ax to the
roots. What are the roots? That *you're* stopping short of God's
standard, accepting (through your eyes and your mind) more than
a hint of immorality in your life.

—adapted from *Every Man's Battle*

But put on the Lord Jesus Christ, and make no provision
for the flesh in regard to its lusts.

ROMANS 13:14, NASB

When you follow the desires of your sinful nature, your
lives will produce these evil results: sexual immorality,
impure thoughts, eagerness for lustful pleasure,...envy,
drunkenness, wild parties, and other kinds of sin. Let me

tell you again, as I have before, that anyone living that sort of life will not inherit the Kingdom of God.

GALATIANS 5:19,21, NLT

I say then: Walk in the Spirit, and you shall not fulfill the lust of the flesh. For the flesh lusts against the Spirit, and the Spirit against the flesh; and these are contrary to one another, so that you do not do the things that you wish.

GALATIANS 5:16-17, NKJV

Beloved, I beg you as aliens and strangers, abstain from fleshly lusts which war against the soul.

1 PETER 2:11, NASB

Put on the full armor of God so that you can take your stand against the devil's schemes. For our struggle is not against flesh and blood, but against the rulers, against the authorities, against the powers of this dark world and against the spiritual forces of evil in the heavenly realms. Therefore put on the full armor of God, so that when the day of evil comes, you may be able to stand your ground, and after you have done everything, to stand. Stand firm then, with the belt of truth buckled around your waist, with the breastplate of righteousness in place, and with your feet fitted with the readiness that comes from the gospel of peace. In addition to all this, take up the shield of faith, with which you can extinguish all the flaming arrows

of the evil one. Take the helmet of salvation and the sword
of the Spirit, which is the word of God.

EPHESIANS 6:11-17, NIV

Sheol (the place of the dead) and Abaddon (the place of
destruction) are never satisfied; so [the lust of] the eyes of
man is never satisfied.

PROVERBS 27:20, AMP

CONTINUE TO FIGHT THE GOOD FIGHT

Fight the good fight for what we believe. Hold tightly to
the eternal life that God has given you, which you have
confessed so well before many witnesses.

1 TIMOTHY 6:12, NLT

Cling tightly to your faith in Christ and always keep your
conscience clear, doing what you know is right. For some
people have disobeyed their consciences and have deliber-
ately done what they knew was wrong.

1 TIMOTHY 1:19, TLB

My son, keep my words
    and treasure up my commandments with you;
keep my commandments and live,
    keep my teachings as the apple of your eye;
bind them on your fingers,

write them on the tablet of your heart.
Say to wisdom, "You are my sister,"
    and call insight your intimate friend;
to preserve you from the loose woman,
    from the adventuress with her smooth words.

PROVERBS 7:1-5, RSV

a battle plan for your marriage

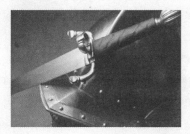

We've known very few men consumed by their marriages, and fewer still consumed by purity, but both are God's desire for you. God's purpose for your marriage is that it parallels Christ's relationship to His church, that you be one with your wife.

Cherishing our wives includes being sexually pure. Are you consumed by this commitment? Consumed enough to live faithfully and to cherish her completely? Consumed enough to stand in harm's way and to eat gravel until God's purposes and your promises are finally established in your land?

If cherishing is anything, it's loving your wife for who she is *this day,* not some other day down the line. It's making allowances for all the surprises and inconsistencies that were hidden until life spun her in its new direction.

Be content with the wife of your youth. If she isn't all you'd hoped for, remember that God graced you with this ewe lamb. Can you make a commitment to cherish her today? If so, let your mind be transformed by the Word.

—adapted from *Every Man's Battle*

YOU'VE MADE A COMMITMENT TO HER AND TO GOD

> LORD, who may dwell in you sanctuary?
> Who may live on your holy hill?
> He…who keeps his oath
> even when it hurts.

> **PSALM 15:1,4, NIV**

And this is his command: to believe in the name of his
Son, Jesus Christ, and to love one another as he commanded us.

1 JOHN 3:23, NIV

A man who makes a vow to the LORD or makes a pledge
under oath must never break it. He must do exactly what
he said he would do.

NUMBERS 30:2, NLT

YOUR COMMITMENT INCLUDES UNWAVERING FAITHFULNESS

You forsake all others on your wedding day. This promise has to
become true in practice and not just in words. You have no right to
think about old girlfriends, and you shouldn't.

—adapted from *Every Man's Battle*

It's harder to make amends with an offended friend than
to capture a fortified city. Arguments separate friends like a
gate locked with iron bars.

PROVERBS 18:19, NLT

Again, you have heard that the ancients were told, "You
shall not make false vows, but shall fulfill our vows to
the LORD."

MATTHEW 5:33, NASB

Thou shalt not commit adultery.

Exodus 20:14, KJV

GOD VIEWS YOUR COVENANT AS UNBREAKABLE

For this cause shall a man leave his father and mother, and cleave to his wife; and they twain shall be one flesh: so then they are no more twain, but one flesh. What therefore God hath joined together, let not man put asunder.

Mark 10:7-9, KJV

Anyone who divorces his wife and marries another woman commits adultery, and the man who marries a divorced woman commits adultery.

Luke 16:18, NIV

Has not the LORD made them one? In flesh and spirit they are his. And why one? Because he was seeking godly offspring. So guard yourself in your spirit, and do not break faith with the wife of your youth.

"I hate divorce," says the LORD God of Israel, "and I hate a man's covering himself with violence as well as with his garment," says the LORD Almighty.

So guard yourself in your spirit, and do not break faith.

Malachi 2:15-16, NIV

YOUR HEART AND BODY BELONG TO HER ALONE

Purifying your eyes and mind is more than a command—it's also a sacrifice. And as you make that sacrifice, as you lay down your desires, blessings will flow. Your spiritual life will experience new joy and power, and your marriage life will blossom as your relationship reaches new heights.

—*Every Man's Battle*

The poor man owned nothing but a little lamb he had worked hard to buy. He raised that little lamb, and it grew up with his children. It ate from the man's own plate and drank from his cup. He cuddled it in his arms like a baby daughter.

2 SAMUEL 12:3, NLT

Rejoice in the wife of your youth. She is a loving doe, a graceful deer. Let her breasts satisfy you always. May you always be captivated by her love.

PROVERBS 5:18-19, NLT

Husbands, love your wives and do not be embittered against them.

COLOSSIANS 3:19, NASB

You know the next commandment pretty well, too: "Don't go to bed with another's spouse." But don't think you've preserved your virtue simply by staying out of bed. Your *heart*

can be corrupted by lust even quicker than your *body*. Those
leering looks you think nobody notices—they also corrupt.

MATTHEW 5:27-28, MSG

But because there is so much sexual immorality, each man
should have his own wife, and each woman should have
her own husband.

The husband should not deprive his wife of sexual
intimacy, which is her right as a married woman, nor
should the wife deprive her husband.

1 CORINTHIANS 7:2-3, NLT

WHAT LOVE IS ALL ABOUT

Remember, the Bible says that God loved us while we were yet sinners. Clearly, loving the unlovely is a foundation of God's character,
and *cherishing* the unlovely is its bedrock. Since Christ died for the
church—the unlovely—and since our marriages should parallel
Christ's relationship to the church, we have no excuse when we
don't cherish our wives. God loved us before we were worthy; we
can do nothing less for our wives.

—*Every Man's Battle*

But God demonstrates his own love for us in this: While
we were still sinners, Christ died for us.

ROMANS 5:8, NIV

In this same way, husbands ought to love their wives as their own bodies. He who loves his wife loves himself. After all, no one ever hated his own body, but he feeds and cares for it, just as Christ does the church—for we are members of his body. "For this reason a man will leave his father and mother and be united to his wife, and the two will become one flesh."

EPHESIANS 5:28-31, NIV

Love is very patient and kind, never jealous or envious, never boastful or proud, never haughty or selfish or rude. Love does not demand its own way. It is not irritable or touchy. It does not hold grudges and will hardly even notice when others do it wrong.

1 CORINTHIANS 13:4-5, TLB

Hatred stirs up strife,
But love covers all sins.

PROVERBS 10:12, NKJV

Love never gives up, never loses faith, is always hopeful, and endures through every circumstance.

1 CORINTHIANS 13:7, NLT

My command is this: Love each other as I have loved you.

JOHN 15:12, NIV

YOUR WIFE'S NEEDS TAKE PRECEDENCE OVER YOUR OWN DESIRES

You husbands must be careful of your wives, being thoughtful of their needs and honoring them as the weaker sex. Remember that you and your wife are partners in receiving God's blessings, and if you don't treat her as you should, your prayers will not get ready answers.

1 PETER 3:7, TLB

Be humble and gentle. Be patient with each other, making allowance for each other's faults because of your love. Always keep yourselves united in the Holy Spirit, and bind yourselves together with peace.

EPHESIANS 4:2-3, NLT

Be kind and compassionate to one another, forgiving each other, just as in Christ God forgave you.

EPHESIANS 4:32, NIV

So, as those who have been chosen of God, holy and beloved, put on a heart of compassion, kindness, humility, gentleness and patience; bearing with one another, and forgiving each other, whoever has a complaint against anyone; just as the Lord forgave you, so also should you.

COLOSSIANS 3:12-13, NASB

dodging enemy fire

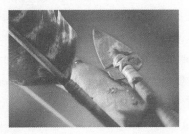

EXAMINE HOW YOU SPEND YOUR TIME

A helpful concept of something to be on the lookout for is the scriptural imagery of "lurking at the door." Maybe your old girlfriend is married now, yet you lurk at her door in your mind, wondering if she misses you, secretly hoping to run into her at the mall.

Or you've been lunching with a group at work, including that beautiful young sales associate, getting so attached that you're depressed whenever she calls in sick. The last time you sent her an e-mail saying, "I missed you today...hope you feel better soon." Innocent, but maybe not so innocent. Or, maybe you've connected with a woman in a chat room, and you imagine what life with her would be like. You're lurking at your neighbor's door.

—adapted from *Every Man's Battle*

If my heart has been enticed by a woman,
    or if I have lurked at my neighbor's door,
then may my wife grind another man's grain,
    and may other men sleep with her.
For that would have been shameful,
    a sin to be judged.

JOB 31:9-11, NIV

So teach us to number our days, that we may get us a heart of wisdom.

PSALM 90:12, AMP

So be careful how you live, not as fools but as those who are wise. Make the most of every opportunity for doing good in these evil days.

EPHESIANS 5:15-16, NLT

GUARD YOUR CONVERSATION

The thoughts of the wicked are an abomination to the LORD,
But the words of the pure are pleasant.

PROVERBS 15:26, NKJV

Words from a wise man's mouth are gracious,
    but a fool is consumed by his own lips.

ECCLESIASTES 10:12, NIV

And the tongue is a fire, a world of iniquity. The tongue is so set among our members that it defiles the whole body, and sets on fire the course of nature; and it is set on fire by hell.

JAMES 3:6, NKJV

Keep your tongue from evil and your lips from speaking deceit.

PSALM 34:13, AMP

Avoid all perverse talk; stay far from corrupt speech.

PROVERBS 4:24, NLT

If anyone considers himself religious and yet does not keep a tight rein on his tongue, he deceives himself and his religion is worthless.

JAMES 1:26, NIV

The fear of the LORD is to hate evil;
Pride and arrogance and the evil way
And the perverse mouth I hate.

PROVERBS 8:13, NKJV

For he that will love life, and see good days, let him refrain his tongue from evil.

1 PETER 3:10, KJV

It would be shameful even to mention here those pleasures of darkness which the ungodly do.

EPHESIANS 5:12, TLB

REMEMBER THAT OTHERS ARE WATCHING

When your son questions what he should watch, what he should do with the pornography other boys show him, or what he should do when that cute girl gets him alone and starts unbuttoning her blouse, what voices will he hear? Will it be your voice, or the voice of his friends? Even his *church* buddies will tell him to go for it. *Your* voice had better be loud and crystal clear because it will probably be the only one whispering, "Flee immorality, son." Your example must be the argument opposing temptation.

—adapted from *Every Man's Battle*

> Conduct yourselves wisely toward outsiders.... Let your speech always be gracious, seasoned with salt, so that you may know how you ought to answer every one.
>
> COLOSSIANS 4:5-6, RSV

> He must also have a good reputation with outsiders, so that he will not fall into disgrace and into the devil's trap.
>
> 1 TIMOTHY 3:7, NIV

> A good name is to be more desired than great wealth, Favor is better than silver and gold.
>
> PROVERBS 22:1, NASB

> A good reputation is more valuable than the most expensive perfume.
>
> ECCLESIASTES 7:1, TLB

PURSUE WISDOM AND COMMON SENSE

> To the man who pleases him, God gives wisdom, knowledge and happiness.
>
> ECCLESIASTES 2:26, NIV

He who trusts in himself is a fool,
>but he who walks in wisdom is kept safe.

PROVERBS 28:26, NIV

Doing wrong is fun for a fool, while wise conduct is a pleasure to the wise.

PROVERBS 10:23, NLT

And the work of righteousness will be peace,
And the service of righteousness, quietness and confidence
>forever.

ISAIAH 32:17, NASB

Wisdom makes one wise man more powerful
>than ten rulers in a city.

ECCLESIASTES 7:19, NIV

Being wise is as good as being rich; in fact, it is better.

ECCLESIASTES 7:11, NLT

Wisdom brightens a man's face
>and changes its hard appearance.

ECCLESIASTES 8:1, NIV

The beginning of wisdom is: Acquire wisdom;
And with all your acquiring, get understanding.

PROVERBS 4:7, NASB

How blessed is the man who finds wisdom
And the man who gains understanding.
For her profit is better than the profit of silver
And her gain better than fine gold.
She is more precious than jewels;
And nothing you desire compares with her.

PROVERBS 3:13-15, NASB

Buy truth, and do not sell it;
buy wisdom, instruction, and understanding.

PROVERBS 23:23, RSV

The godly give good advice, but fools are destroyed by
their lack of common sense.

PROVERBS 10:21, NLT

The mind of the prudent acquires knowledge,
And the ear of the wise seeks knowledge.

PROVERBS 18:15, NASB

The discerning heart seeks knowledge,
but the mouth of a fool feeds on folly.

PROVERBS 15:14, NIV

A house is built by wisdom and becomes strong through
good sense.

PROVERBS 24:3, NLT

So I decided to compare wisdom and folly, and anyone else would come to the same conclusions I [King Solomon] did. Wisdom is of more value than foolishness, just as light is better than darkness. For the wise person sees, while the fool is blind.

ECCLESIASTES 2:12-14, NLT

Wisdom or money can get you almost anything, but it's important to know that only wisdom can save your life.

ECCLESIASTES 7:12, NLT

It is better to be criticized by a wise person than to be praised by a fool! Indeed, a fool's laughter is quickly gone, like thorns crackling in a fire.

ECCLESIASTES 7:5-6, NLT

KEEP YOUR EYES ON THE PRIZE

In transforming your mind, you'll be taking an active, conscious role in capturing rogue thoughts, but in the long run, the mind will wash itself and will begin to work naturally for you and your purity by capturing such thoughts. With the eyes bouncing away from sexual images and the mind policing itself, your defenses will grow incredibly strong.

—Every Man's Battle

My son, let them not vanish from your sight;
Keep sound wisdom and discretion,
So they will be life to your soul
And adornment to your neck.
Then you will walk in your way securely
And your foot will not stumble.
When you lie down, you will not be afraid;
When you lie down, your sleep will be sweet.
Do not be afraid of sudden fear
Nor of the onslaught of the wicked when it comes;
For the LORD will be your confidence
And will keep your foot from being caught.

PROVERBS 3:21-26, NASB

My son, do not forget my teaching.
But let your heart keep my commandments;
For length of days and years of life
And peace they will add to you.

PROVERBS 3:1-2, NASB

How beautiful your sandaled feet,
    O prince's daughter!
Your graceful legs are like jewels,
    the work of a craftsman's hands.
Your navel is a rounded goblet
    that never lacks blended wine.

Your waist is a mound of wheat
   encircled by lilies.
Your breasts are like two fawns,
   twins of a gazelle.
Your neck is like an ivory tower.
Your eyes are the pools of Heshbon
   by the gate of Bath Rabbim.
Your nose is like the tower of Lebanon
   looking toward Damascus.
Your head crowns you like Mount Carmel.
   Your hair is like royal tapestry;
   the king is held captive by its tresses.
How beautiful you are and how pleasing,
   O love, with your delights!
Your stature is like that of the palm,
   and your breasts like clusters of fruit.
I said, "I will climb the palm tree;
   I will take hold of its fruit."
May your breasts be like the clusters of the vine,
   the fragrance of your breath like apples,
   and your mouth like the best wine.

SONG OF SONGS 7:1-9, NIV

Before long, you will feel a new light and lightness in your soul.
Along with inner peace comes an outer peace that affects your
daily life.

—adapted from *Every Man's Battle*

He that walketh uprightly walketh surely: but he that per-
verteth his ways shall be known.

PROVERBS 10:9, KJV

The wages of the righteous bring them life,
   but the income of the wicked brings them
      punishment.

PROVERBS 10:16, NIV

The curse of the LORD is on the house of the wicked, but
his blessing is on the home of the upright.

PROVERBS 3:33, NLT

Praise the LORD.
Blessed is the man who fears the LORD,
   who finds great delight in his commands.
His children will be mighty in the land;
   the generation of the upright will be blessed.

PSALM 112:1-2, NIV

The righteous man leads a blameless life;
   blessed are his children after him.

PROVERBS 20:7, NIV

But as for you [Titus], promote the kind of living that
reflects right teaching. Teach the older men to exercise self-
control, to be worthy of respect, and to live wisely. They

must have strong faith and be filled with love and
patience.

TITUS 2:1-2, NLT

For I am confident of this very thing, that He who began a
good work in you will perfect it until the day of Christ Jesus.

PHILIPPIANS 1:6, NASB

CONSIDER THE BENEFITS OF FEARING GOD

Love the LORD your God with all your heart and with all
your soul and with all your strength. These commandments that I give you today are to be upon your hearts.

DEUTERONOMY 6:5-6, NIV

He who is steadfast in righteousness will live,
    but he who pursues evil will die.

PROVERBS 11:19, RSV

Fear of the LORD gives life, security, and protection from
harm.

PROVERBS 19:23, NLT

In the way of righteousness is life,
And in its pathway there is no death.

PROVERBS 12:28, NASB

The fear of the LORD is a fountain of life,
To turn one away from the snares of death.

PROVERBS 14:27, NKJV

Do not let your heart envy sinners,
But live in the fear of the LORD always.

PROVERBS 23:17, NASB

For while bodily training is of some value, godliness is of
value in every way, as it holds promise for the present life
and also for the life to come.

1 TIMOTHY 4:8, RSV

The path of the upright leads away from evil; whoever follows that path is safe.

PROVERBS 16:17, NLT

When the storm has swept by, the wicked are gone,
    but the righteous stand firm forever.

PROVERBS 10:25, NIV

The prospect of the righteous is joy,
    but the hopes of the wicked come to nothing.
The way of the LORD is a refuge for the
        righteous,
    but it is the ruin of those who do evil.

The righteous will never be uprooted,
> but the wicked will not remain in the land.

> > PROVERBS 10:28-30, NIV

For the perverse person is an abomination to the LORD,
But His secret counsel is with the upright.

> > PROVERBS 3:32, NKJV

Don't worry about the wicked.
> Don't envy those who do wrong.
For like grass, they soon fade away.
> Like springtime flowers, they soon wither.
Trust in the LORD and do good.
> Then you will live safely in the land and prosper.

> > PSALM 37:1-3, NLT

The righteousness of the upright will deliver them,
But the unfaithful will be caught by their lust.

> > PROVERBS 11:6, NKJV

God rescues good men from danger while letting the
wicked fall into it.

> > PROVERBS 11:8, TLB

The desire of the righteous ends only in good;
> the expectation of the wicked in wrath.

> > PROVERBS 11:23, RSV

He that followeth after righteousness and mercy findeth life, righteousness, and honour.

PROVERBS 21:21, KJV

A wicked man hardens his face,
But as for the upright, he establishes his way.

PROVERBS 21:29, NKJV

the ultimate secret
to overcoming sin

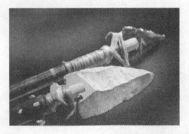

The key to victory in the battle for sexual purity lies in the fact that, as believers, we have the Holy Spirit constantly at our side to help us fight our battles. Without His presence, we have little hope of overcoming the pressures of the world. Now is the perfect time to examine your heart and be sure that you have truly entrusted your heart and life to God, guaranteeing for yourself a Companion who will fight with you and for you.

In Scripture, the "Roman Road" teaches us that everyone has sinned (Romans 3:23), the penalty for our sin is death (Romans 6:23), Jesus Christ died for our sins (Romans 5:8), and to be forgiven for our sins, we must believe and confess that Jesus is Lord, because salvation only comes through Jesus Christ (Romans 10:8-10).

Have you walked the truths of the Roman Road? If not, you can come to know Christ right now by reading and confessing this set of verses. When you trust in Christ, you will spend eternity with Him.

THE ROMAN ROAD

For all have sinned; all fall short of God's glorious standard.

ROMANS 3:23, NLT

Salvation that comes from trusting Christ—which is the message we preach—is already within easy reach. In fact, the Scriptures say, "The message is close at hand; it is on your lips and in your heart."

For if you confess with your mouth that Jesus is Lord and believe in your heart that God raised him from the dead, you will be saved. For it is by believing in your heart that you are made right with God, and it is by confessing with your mouth that you are saved.

ROMANS 10:8-10, NLT

For the wages of sin is death, but the free gift of God is eternal life through Christ Jesus our Lord.

ROMANS 6:23, NLT

But God showed his great love for us by sending Christ to die for us while we were still sinners.

ROMANS 5:8, NLT

THE PROMISE OF THE HOLY SPIRIT

Those who obey God's commandments live in fellowship with him, and he with them. And we know he lives in us because the Holy Spirit lives in us.

1 JOHN 3:24, NLT

But you are not like that. You are controlled by your new nature if you have the Spirit of God living in you. (And remember that if anyone doesn't have the Spirit of Christ living him, he is not a Christian at all.)

ROMANS 8:9, TLB

And I will put my Spirit in you and move you to follow my decrees and be careful to keep my laws.

EZEKIEL 36:27, NIV

For his Holy Spirit speaks to us deep in our hearts and tells us that we are God's children.

ROMANS 8:16, NLT

We know that we live in him and he in us, because he has given us of his Spirit.

1 JOHN 4:13, NIV

For as many as are led by the Spirit of God, these are sons of God.

ROMANS 8:14, NKJV

ready your weapons,
raise your shield

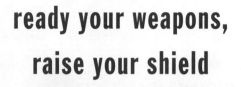

What about you, in your battle with impure eyes and mind? What's your alternative to fighting?

To stay ensnared and die spiritually.

- How long are you going to stay sexually impure?
- How long will you rob your wife sexually?
- How long will you stunt the growth of oneness with your wife, a oneness you promised her years ago?

—adapted from *Every Man's Battle*

A TIME TO SURRENDER TO GOD'S PLAN

God has made everything beautiful for its own time. He has planted eternity in the human heart, but even so, people cannot see the whole scope of God's work from beginning to end.

ECCLESIASTES 3:11, NLT

Nevertheless, God's solid foundation stands firm, sealed with this inscription: "The Lord knows those who are his," and, "Everyone who confesses the name of the Lord must turn away from wickedness."

2 TIMOTHY 2:19, NIV

Today I have given you the choice between life and death, between blessings and curses.... Oh, that you would choose life, that you and your descendants might live!

DEUTERONOMY 30:19, NLT

There is a time for everything,
a season for every activity under heaven.
A time to be born and a time to die.
A time to plant and a time to harvest.
A time to kill and a time to heal.
A time to tear down and a time to rebuild.
A time to cry and a time to laugh.
A time to grieve and a time to dance.
A time to scatter stones and a time to gather stones.
A time to embrace and a time to turn away.
A time to search and a time to lose.
A time to keep and a time to throw away.
A time to tear and a time to mend.
A time to be quiet and a time to speak up.
A time to love and a time to hate.
A time for war and a time for peace.

ECCLESIASTES 3:1-8, NLT

A TIME TO FIGHT

Fight the good fight of the faith. Take hold of the eternal life to which you were called when you made your good confession in the presence of many witnesses.

1 TIMOTHY 6:12, NIV

Put on God's whole armor [the armor of a heavy-armed soldier which God supplies], that you may be able successfully to stand up against [all] the strategies and the deceits of the devil.

EPHESIANS 6:11, AMP

But let us who live in the light keep sober, protected by the armor of faith and love, and wearing as our helmet the happy hope of salvation.

1 THESSALONIANS 5:8, TLB

He will cover you with His pinions,
And under His wings you may seek refuge;
His faithfulness is a shield and bulwark.

PSALM 91:4, NASB

For surely, O LORD, you bless the righteous;
    you surround them with your favor as with a shield.

PSALM 5:12, NIV

We depend on the LORD alone to save us.
    Only he can help us, protecting us like a shield.

PSALM 33:20, NLT

For Jehovah God is our Light and our Protector. He gives us grace and glory. No good thing will he withhold from those who walk along his paths.

PSALM 84:11, TLB

every man's battle
workshops

from New Life Ministries

New Life Ministries receives hundreds of calls every month from Christian men who are struggling to stay pure in the midst of daily challenges to their sexual integrity and from pastors who are looking for guidance in how to keep fragile marriages from falling apart all around them.

As part of our commitment to equip individuals to win these battles, New Life Ministries has developed biblically based workshops directly geared to answer these needs. These workshops are held several times per year around the country.

- Our workshops **for men** are structured to equip men with the tools necessary to maintain sexual integrity and enjoy healthy, productive relationships.

- Our workshops **for church leaders** are targeted to help pastors and men's ministry leaders develop programs to help families being attacked by this destructive addiction.

Some comments from previous workshop attendees:

"An awesome, life-changing experience. Awesome teaching, teacher, content and program." —DAVE

"God has truly worked a great work in me since the EMB workshop. I am fully confident that with God's help, I will be restored in my ministry position. Thank you for your concern. I realize that this is a battle, but I now have the weapons of warfare as mentioned in Ephesians 6:10, and I am using them to gain victory!" —KEN

"It's great to have a workshop you can confidently recommend to anyone without hesitation, knowing that it is truly life changing. Your labors are not in vain!" —DR. BRAD STENBERG, Pasadena, CA

If sexual temptation is threatening your marriage or your church, please call **1-800-NEW-LIFE** to speak with one of our specialists.

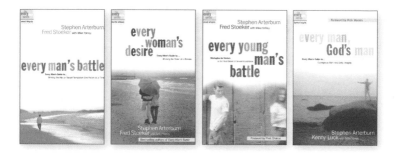
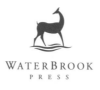